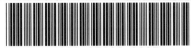
100 Questions & Answers

About Stroke

A Lahey Clinic Guide

Kinan K. Hreib, MD, PhD

Director of Vascular Neurology
Department of Neurology
Lahey Clinic
Burlington, MA

JONES AND BARTLETT PUBLISHERS

Sudbury, Massachusetts

BOSTON   TORONTO   LONDON   SINGAPORE

World Headquarters

Jones and Bartlett Publishers
40 Tall Pine Drive
Sudbury, MA 01776
978-443-5000
info@jbpub.com
www.jbpub.com

Jones and Bartlett Publishers
Canada
6339 Ormindale Way
Mississauga, Ontario L5V 1J2
CANADA

Jones and Bartlett Publishers
International
Barb House, Barb Mews
London W6 7PA
UK

Jones and Bartlett's books and products are available through most bookstores and online booksellers. To contact Jones and Bartlett Publishers directly, call 800-832-0034, fax 978-443-8000, or visit our website, www.jbpub.com.

Substantial discounts on bulk quantities of Jones and Bartlett's publications are available to corporations, professional associations, and other qualified organizations. For details and specific discount information, contact the special sales department at Jones and Bartlett via the above contact information or send an email to specialsales@jbpub.com.

The authors, editor, and publisher have made every effort to provide accurate information. However, they are not responsible for errors, omissions, or for any outcomes related to the use of the contents of this book and take no responsibility for the use of the products and procedures described. Treatments and side effects described in this book may not be applicable to all people; likewise, some people may require a dose or experience a side effect that is not described herein. Drugs and medical devices are discussed that may have limited availability controlled by the Food and Drug Administration (FDA) for use only in a research study or clinical trial. Research, clinical practice, and government regulations often change the accepted standard in this field. When consideration is being given to use of any drug in the clinical setting, the health care provider or reader is responsible for determining FDA status of the drug, reading the package insert, and reviewing prescribing information for the most up-to-date recommendations on dose, precautions, and contraindications, and determining the appropriate usage for the product. This is especially important in the case of drugs that are new or seldom used.

Library of Congress Cataloging-in-Publication Data
Hreib, Kinan K.
 100 questions and answers about stroke : a Lahey Clinic guide / Kinan K. Hreib.
   p. cm.
 Includes index.
 ISBN-13: 978-0-7637-5070-1 (pbk. : alk. paper)
 ISBN-10: 0-7637-5070-0
 1. Cerebrovascular disease--Miscellanea. 2. Cerebrovascular disease--Popular works. I. Title. II. Title: One hundred questions and answers about stroke.
 RC388.5.H72 2008
 616.8'1--dc22
                          200702140
6048

Production Credits
Executive Editor: Christopher Davis
Production Director: Amy Rose
Associate Production Editor: Rachel Rossi
Associate Editor: Kathy Richardson
Associate Marketing Manager: Rebecca Wasley

Manufacturing Buyer: Therese Connell
Composition: Appingo
Cover Design: Jonathan Ayotte
Printing and Binding: Malloy, Inc.
Cover Printing: Malloy, Inc.

Printed in the United States of America
11 10 09 08   10 9 8 7 6 5 4 3 2 1

I dedicate this book to
Marina, Katherine, and Alexander.

CONTENTS

Last year, at the age of 38, I had a stroke. I thought strokes happened to old people; I was young and healthy with two young children. One day after a short jog, I developed a headache. I had had headaches before, but this new headache was different: It was on the right side of my head and more severe than usual. I was concerned, but because I have had headaches that subsided before, I had a sense of false comfort. I kept saying to myself, this headache will go away like all the others. I should have listened to my inside voice telling me something was wrong.

I should have listened, but I decided to find a more comforting explanation. The next morning the headache continued, becoming more severe. I took some Tylenol and drove the kids to school, as I usually do. The children knew something was not right. My daughter asked me if I was feeling okay. Later that day I collapsed to the floor, not able to move the left side of my body. I did not know what happened. I had a feeling that it had something to do with my headache. I tried to get up to reach the phone. All I could think about was who was going to get the children from school, feed them dinner, and help them with their homework. I crawled slowly on the floor until I reached the telephone, pulled the telephone down to the floor, and called for help. The emergency medical technicians arrived within 10 minutes. During those 10 minutes I called my husband and told him about the problems I was having; he was having a hard time understanding me, and I realized I had a problem with my speech. He knew there was something wrong.

I was taken to the emergency room of a local hospital, and my husband, Tom, arrived half an hour later. I was confused and didn't know what had happened, and my husband was clearly panicked, trying to find a doctor to talk to, wanting answers quickly. I could hear my husband screaming at the nurses and doctors; he was tearful and scared. I tried to move. I wanted to get up and walk away from this nightmare, but I couldn't. I started crying, and my left arm and leg were not moving. I felt helpless. I had a great life and family and I was healthy. What had happened? Why me, God? Why me? Did I do something wrong to deserve this? Can somebody help me?

I heard sounds in the background. People were running around, some talking to me and others not. Someone was taking blood from my arm while another person was putting a needle in my other arm. I knew they were talking to me and I could hear them, but in my state of absolute panic I could not focus. I tried to talk; my speech was slow and difficult to understand. I looked in the eyes of the doctors and nurses for answers. I wanted to make sure they saw me. I was trying to read their faces. What is going on with me? Please tell me. The doctors were asking questions about my symptoms. I tried to answer, hoping that my answers would help them with the diagnosis. One of them finally said he thought I was having a stroke. I am not sure I fully comprehended what he said to me. As they wheeled me to the scanner, I began thinking of how a stroke could affect me. I have seen people with stroke; some were in bad shape. Some could not talk or eat on their own; some could not walk or use their arm. What's going to happen to my children? Did I cause the stroke? What's going to happen to me? Please, God, give me another chance.

My husband followed me to the scanner. I could see his tears, but I don't think he talked—he probably didn't know what to say. The scan took less than 5 minutes. I was hoping the doctors were wrong and that when the scan was done I could just walk off the stretcher and out of the emergency room, back to my comfortable home with my children. I finally asked Tom about the kids. He told me they were with their grandmother and were okay. One of the doctors walked in to tell me that the CT was normal. For a few seconds I felt relieved that there was no stroke. But the doctor then explained that the CT may not detect the stroke and that he and his team of other doctors believed that I had experienced a stroke. Before I could ask whether they could do something to help me, the doctor was telling me about a drug that could possibly help my stroke. My mind was racing; I don't think I heard everything the doctor said.

Now I know that he talked to me and my husband about t-PA. He told us the drug was not effective in all cases and that it may kill me. For a moment I thought the doctor had the answer, but even in my shocked state I could tell the treatment was risky and that the doctor was uncertain about the treatment. I later learned that giving t-PA is not straightforward. I wanted something to help me; I really wanted to go back home; I did not want my kids to see me like this. Tom believed that the drug was risky, but I said I wanted to receive it. I received the medication while in the emergency room, but my symptoms did not go away. I felt desperate, but I was also very tired. I fell asleep until the next morning.

The next day my husband and my children came to visit. My daughter cried and looked terrified. My son was composed but very uncomfortable. He did not want to hug me and sat far away from the bed. After my family left I felt lonely. I wished there were someone with me just to tell me that it was going to be okay. A whole bunch of doctors came in to talk to me. They asked me to do things with my left arm, but I couldn't. However, my left leg was moving. I smiled at the first glimmer of hope, a small victory perhaps. I wanted some feedback from the doctors, and one of them said the movement was a good sign. I had not had anything to eat in more than 24 hours, but I wasn't hungry. The doctor told me they would do more tests to figure out what caused the stroke, and they would also test my swallowing before I was allowed to eat. For the next few days I stayed in the hospital. I wanted to leave, but I knew I could not take care of myself or my children. I started feeling desperate again. I was hoping that I would regain strength and be back to normal by now, but only my leg was moving. I didn't even know if my leg was strong enough to stand on. My swallowing was fine, so I was allowed to eat. I must have been hungry because the hospital food tasted good. My family visited every day, and by the third day my son gave me a hug and sat next to me, stroking my head. From that moment on I knew that no matter what deficits I had that I was still loved and that the stroke had not taken away my motherhood or who I was to my family.

Finally, I was discharged to a rehabilitation hospital where I stayed for almost 2 months. During that time I worked hard to stand up with help and then independently. Strength in my left arm slowly improved, but my hand remained weak. My speech went back to normal. While at the rehabilitation hospital I was treated for depression and for some pain that I developed in my left shoulder. My husband, family, and friends visited me every day. I got to know my family, and my family got to know me in a different way. I found my family to be very supportive, and I saw the compassion of strangers. Many other people with stroke, young and old, became my friends. Age didn't seem to be an obstacle: We shared the same problems, we had the same pain, we all walked "funny," and some talked like drunks. Some days were more depressing than others, but I knew that I had a family waiting for me. The 2 months in rehabilitation were the longest 2 months of my life, and the most painful, but at the end of it, I felt more alive. Humpty Dumpty was back together, scarred but definitely alive.

My self-employed husband stopped working for almost 3 months. We depleted our savings and had to borrow money. Now, almost 1 year after the stroke I am still not back to normal, but I have stopped feeling sorry for myself. I force myself to get out of bed every day. I get tired quickly, but I take a nap and then do more. I tried jogging again but the spastic leg and joint pains made this difficult. I am now a great swimmer. Being in the pool takes the weight off my joints, and I can still get a workout without too much pain.

I know that I have a purpose. I speak to support groups and anyone who is willing to listen about my stroke. I tell people who suffered from stroke not to give up. I did not realize how slow my recovery would be, and I did not realize what can happen to the body after a stroke or how my stroke was going to affect people around me. My immediate family went through a period of grief at my apparent loss. I grieved too for my lost self, but my family and I learned to like the new me. I have a different perspective on life. My life was turned upside down in only a few hours and a year later I am still not right-side-up, but I no longer think of the events as a big tragedy. I don't know what made me feel better and start to recover, but I know that my family gave me a purpose to work hard and recover.

—SH

This book is intended as a guide for patients and families who have suffered from stroke or those who are interested in reviewing the diagnosis and treatment of cerebrovascular disease. It is difficult to provide a comprehensive understanding of all the issues related to stroke in this book, but I hope the information is helpful in understanding some aspects of the diagnosis and the available treatments for this disease. In writing this book and in attempting to explain the complexity of stroke, I realized that my task could be hindered by my biases and my own experiences. Therefore I tried to find literature that is pertinent to each topic, interpret the findings or recommendations, and then make some practical comments. As you will see throughout this book, some studies to help guide treatment of certain diseases often fail to address some aspects of disease management, whereas other studies provide data that beg for additional clarity. Ultimately, decisions regarding treatment must not be done without the use of known literature, the physician's own experience, and an understanding between the patient and the physician about the risk and benefits of a given treatment.

An important aspect of treatment in medicine is guidelines. Guidelines are intended to standardize some aspects of medical care to create consistency, streamline the evaluation, and expedite treatment. Although specific guidelines are truly intended to help "guide" the care of well-defined medical problems, such as pneumonia or congestive heart failure, guidelines for stroke by necessity have to be more general, because the disease entity is more complex, the diagnosis of stroke is not always obvious, and other conditions can mimic stroke. Although it is easy to understand the impetus behind the implementation of guidelines, the decision-making process of physicians requires information and input that may change over the course of treatment, rendering guidelines useless in some cases. Furthermore, many medical conditions do not lend themselves to guidelines. Under those circumstances evaluation, diagnosis, and treatment depend on the physician's own experience and knowledge. Critics of guidelines are concerned that guidelines create the perception that all of medicine can be distilled to predetermined tests and treatments. As a result, relying on guidelines alone limits the flexibility of care, may hinder a change in the direction of care if necessary, and further compounds rigid thinking about certain medical conditions. Therefore guidelines are simply a guide to treatment, but, alone are not sufficient to treat patients. Guidelines do not obviate the need for constant input from the medical staff.

In treating complicated medical conditions, such as a stroke, physicians need to have basic knowledge that allows them to diagnose the condition, to perform appropriate tests, and to design a treatment. The process that allows these abilities to develop is shaped by many different elements, including book knowledge, exposure to the literature, mentorship, experience, and critical thinking. The training of physicians is rigorous and highly regimented, some may even say inflexible. When physicians complete their formal training, their exposure to patient care has generally been fairly scripted by their mentors. The biases of these mentors inevitably become part of the early understanding of the physician's approach to disease processes and treatment. Fostering inquisitiveness in young physicians is important but may be difficult to accomplish. Inquisitiveness is an especially important characteristic when we are faced with complicated medical conditions. Unfortunately, the time constraints that physicians are under makes intellectual contemplation about a complicated case even more challenging. Time constraints in the office, and overflowing emergency rooms, prevent physicians from spending the required time to foster trust with patients and obtain all the necessary information. Although common neurological problems that present with "classic" symptoms are often diagnosed and managed appropriately, common problems presenting with unusual symptoms may be the most missed type of condition. The obstacles of reaching a diagnosis are sometimes difficult to pinpoint. Physicians may have some biases that prevent them from establishing trust with the patient. Sometimes the patient is unable to give a good history. Seeing the patient over an extended period of time and using eyewitnesses may be necessary, although it is very time consuming and sometimes not possible to accomplish.

It is ideal to establish a professional relationship between the patient and the physician that fosters trust. Conflicts between patients and physicians sometimes emerge and may get in the way of establishing a trusting relationship.

Conflicts arise because of perceptions that the patient is too demanding or that the physician is uncaring. Patients often expect that a specialist has all the answers and that a cure must exist somewhere. Patients are constantly seeking the latest in treatment or imaging, basing much of that interest on advertisement. Physicians, on the other hand, are by nature "conservative." They are often hesitant to embrace new treatments and technologies. Physicians believe there are many valid reasons for delaying implementation of new treatments, including the lack of scientific data, as some studies are poorly designed. Or that the data show only marginal benefit and therefore are not likely to make a difference in most patients. Furthermore, as serious side effects of well-studied drugs emerge once released to the market, one has to wonder about the accuracy of some of these studies or whether the studies have specific design flaws that limit their interpretation. Understanding some of these issues surrounding medical care will help promote a more productive and understanding relationship between the patient and the physician.

The concepts in the book have been simplified to help the reader understand the basic pathophysiology of strokes. Furthermore, each section is organized to give the reader a general review of the condition, current diagnostic and treatment options, and controversies. The book was written with the understanding that many patients already have a fairly good understanding of medical issues. Access to medical opinions and material on the Internet has made many patients much more aware of the issues surrounding their own medical problems. As a result, in writing this book, I took into consideration that many patients understand medicine now better than they ever did and that "dumbing down" the book would truly be an insult to the intellect of our patients. This book was not intended as a cookbook, and patients should take into consideration the complex nature of medicine as well as the constantly evolving concepts in diagnosis and treatments.

Epidemiology

Stroke affects over 700,000 patients per year, with an average of 35% of stroke survivors suffering from partial or complete disability. Over 30% of stroke survivors suffer from cognitive decline, 13% die from another stroke, and 30% die from heart-related problems in the next 5 years after the initial stroke. The largest portion of the population affected by stroke is over the age of 65. Senior citizens are the fastest growing group of the population in the United States. By 2030, it is estimated that the number of senior citizens will grow to 55 million. The direct cost of taking care of patients with acute stroke is over 40 billion dollars per year. Often, care for stroke survivors continues after the acute hospitalization, with substantial contributions from family, friends, and the community. The cost of such services is unknown but is likely to be substantial. Therefore, stroke places a significant burden on the entire society as reflected by the cost of stroke care, loss of income, and loss of productivity. As the population ages, we are likely to see a large demand for medical services, with elderly patients using three times the resources as younger individuals. This issue is likely to create significant generational conflicts as limited resources and increasing concerns about health care cost and rising poverty become important issues to discuss.

PART ONE

The Basics

What is a stroke?

What is a transient ischemic attack (TIA)?

What is the difference between transient
ischemic attack and stroke?

More . . .

1. What is a stroke?

A **stroke** is damage to the brain or the spinal cord as a result of an abnormality in an artery or vein. There are two major types of strokes: ischemic and hemorrhagic. **Ischemic strokes** are caused by critical decrease of blood flow to parts of the brain, causing the death of brain cells. **Hemorrhagic strokes** are caused by a break in the wall of the artery, causing spillage of blood inside the brain or around the brain. This book does not discuss strokes of the spinal cord.

In the United States it is estimated that approximately 700,000 strokes occur per year. The incidence of ischemic stroke is approximately 300 per 100,000 individuals. The incidence of ischemic stroke in African-Americans is substantially higher than in whites. Hemorrhagic strokes account for approximately 10% of all strokes, with a higher predilection in African-Americans and those of Asian descent. The racial and ethnic differences in stroke incidence are a major finding that deserves further investigations.

An interesting fact about ischemic strokes is that they often occur between 10:00 AM to noon. It is believed that strokes caused by an evolving clot in the large arteries leading to the brain occur at night when the circulation is less active. On the other hand, **embolic strokes**, such as strokes from irregular heartbeat, like atrial fibrillation, occur with activities.

When I presented at the hospital, I knew that my condition was serious, but I never thought about stroke. Then I was being rushed down a hallway on a gurney to get a CAT scan after vomiting, and the nurse asked me to grab his fingers. Suddenly I could no longer see or move. It was at this point that I asked if I was having a stroke. To this day, I find it odd that I would pose this question, as I was a healthy 37-year-old, who took long power walks at lunch. There was no family history of stroke. In fact, I didn't know anyone personally who had had a stroke, and was clueless as to the

---

A stroke is damage to the brain or the spinal cord as a result of an abnormality in an artery or vein.

Stroke

Any damage to the brain or spinal cord caused by obstruction or damage to artery or vein.

Ischemic stroke

Damage to the brain related to obstruction of artery.

Hemorrhagic stroke

Damage to the brain related to bleeding.

An interesting fact about ischemic strokes is that they often occur between 10:00 am to noon.

---

symptoms of stroke. To instinctively be aware that I was having a stroke demonstrates the power of intuition.

2. What is a transient ischemic attack (TIA)?

The definition implies that there are no permanent neurological symptoms or damage to the brain as a result of decreased blood flow. In the past, neurologists believed that symptoms lasting less than 24 hours should be classified as transient ischemic attack. With better imaging, such as **magnetic resonance imaging (MRI)**, it turned out that many patients who had symptoms for less than 24 hours had evidence of stroke on the MRI. Therefore the definition was changed to include only patients who have symptoms for 1 hour or less. But in spite of this more strict definition, it has been shown that a significant number of patients show evidence of a stroke on the MRI, albeit without evidence of neurological deficits. Differentiating between "transient ischemic attack" and stroke is not as important as it may seem to some, because both conditions suggest a problem with the blood flow and both conditions require immediate attention.

The incidence of **transient ischemic attack (TIA)** is estimated at 202 per 100,000 individuals. In younger individuals the incidence is around 50 per 100,000 and at the age of 75 the incidence increases to around 680 per 100,000. In the older group gender differences are seen, with approximately 100 fewer transient ischemic attacks in women than in men. The incidence of transient ischemic attacks preceding a stroke is estimated to be approximately 10%. This relatively low incidence of transient ischemic attacks in stroke is likely related to multiple factors, including the underlying pathology, such as carotid artery disease versus cardiac source. But it is also likely that patients simply under-report transient ischemic attack or simply do not appreciate the symptoms of transient ischemic attack.

Embolic stroke

This refers to stroke from blood clots or other debris that has traveled from another source before it finally gets lodged in an artery, causing stroke.

Magnetic resonance imaging (MRI)

Uses a large magnet instead of an x-ray to see the inside of the body.

Transient ischemic attack (TIA)

Transient neurological symptoms related to disruption of blood flow to certain parts of the brain.

The Basics

Because symptoms of transient ischemia deserve immediate attention, the individual should contact the primary care physician or get to the emergency room immediately. If the individual does not have allergies to aspirin he or she should take one adult-size aspirin. Although the symptoms may resolve promptly, there is still a significant risk for stroke. Studies on the risk of heart attack and vascular death after transient ischemic attack and ischemic stroke revealed that the risk of stroke after transient ischemic attack was 9.5% at 90 days and 14.5% at 1 year. The risk of combined stroke, heart attack, or death was 21.8% at 1 year. Therefore a transient ischemic attack is a serious condition that needs to be addressed promptly. A transient ischemic attack is also is a warning sign of coexisting vascular disease, including heart attacks.

Transient ischemia-like symptoms can occur with tumors, bleeding inside the brain, and inflammatory conditions of the brain. The cause of the symptoms needs to be determined for the correct treatment to be instituted.

3. What is the difference between transient ischemic attack and stroke?

The diagnosis of transient ischemic attack is based solely on symptom onset and resolution of those symptoms in less than an hour. But imaging of the brain may show changes consistent with stroke in a location relevant to the symptoms. Therefore our definitions of transient ischemic attacks are based on the relationship between clinical symptoms and imaging studies. In the past and before MRI, a **computed tomography (CT)**, another type of scan, was the only imaging technology available to look at the brain. CTs are good at revealing bleeding inside the brain, but small nonbleeding strokes, referred to as infarcts, are often missed on the CT. Even large infarcts may be missed acutely on the CT. A small clot that blocks flow to one artery and then disintegrates may still result in some damage to brain structures but without causing ongoing symptoms. The amount of ongoing symptoms after

Computed tomography (CT)

A fancy x-ray machine that takes pictures of the brain.

vascular damage in the brain depends on the location of the damage. Although, generally, larger strokes can cause more symptoms, small strokes in strategic areas can be devastating. More sophisticated imaging of the brain with MRI can provide more details about areas of damage in patients with transient ischemia. A sequence on MRI, known as diffusion sequence, can be extremely sensitive in detecting cellular damage caused by stroke and possibly other processes. Comparing diffusion sequences to other sequences on MRI allows physicians to determine when the damage occurred. In some cases, changes noted on the diffusion images reverse relatively quickly. Under most circumstances, the changes resolve after a few weeks. More recent studies using "diffusion" MRI show that 50% of patients with transient ischemic attacks have in fact suffered from a stroke (i.e., permanent damage to part of the brain). Therefore it seems that our definitions of transient ischemic attacks are still evolving. The difference between transient ischemia and stroke is simply the presence or absence of on-going symptoms. The zealously by which we need to find the cause of the symptoms should be the same. Transient ischemic attacks and stroke are part of the same disease process.

4. What are the major causes of stroke?

Much of our understanding of this topic is continuing to evolve. Population studies have suggested that approximately 15% of all strokes are related to diseased arteries in the neck or the skull; approximately 15% are related to small arteries in the deep parts of the brain, causing "lacunar" strokes; approximately 30% are from a cardiac source and approximately 30% to 40% are of unknown etiology. Other studies attempting to address similar questions suggest that the percentage of strokes with unknown etiology is much smaller, if we consider smoking, hypertension, diabetes, estrogen replacement therapy, migraines, and underlying clotting disorders as important stand-alone risks for strokes.

More recent studies using sophisticated imaging of the brain, such as "diffusion" MRI show that 50% of patients with transient ischemic attacks have in fact suffered from a stroke (i.e., permanent damage to part of the brain).

The Basics

5. How does a CT help with the diagnosis of stroke?

Computed tomography or CT is a fancy x-ray machine with multiple x-ray tubes arranged in a circle. The circle is a donut-shaped hole that the head or body is actually placed in. Inside the donut the tubes spin and take multiple images that the computer then translates into pictures. The CT uses actual radiation to obtain these pictures. The advantage of the CT is that it is readily available and is fast. The major uses of the CT are to detect acute blood in the brain or significant stroke that is at least several hours old. The obvious drawback then is that fresh strokes may not be seen or easily appreciated and older blood, a few days old, may not be detected. Furthermore, subtle changes in areas in the bottom part of the brain, where the skull is thick, or even near sharp skull areas may not be appreciated.

Sometimes, a CT of the brain is done with contrast. Contrast is a substance injected in the vein that then circulates to the brain and may help define abnormal structures such as tumors. Some people may be allergic to contrast. The incidence of allergy to contrast ranges from 2% to 12%. Patients who are allergic to contrast should not receive this material, or if contrast is absolutely necessary, then steroids and Benadryl may be given before the contrast is administered. However, pretreatment does not completely eliminate the risk of a reaction. Some patients may also have compromised kidney function, and those patients should be cleared by their doctor before receiving the contrast.

6. How does an MRI help with the diagnosis of stroke?

Magnetic resonance imaging or MRI is the most sophisticated technology to provide detailed images of the brain. The MRI does not use any radiation, unlike computer tomography or CT. The principle of MRI technology is primarily based on detecting magnetic signal from molecules in the tissue. Most of the signal comes from the abundant hydrogen molecule. But other molecules have different magnetic characteristics. The MRI can pick up these magnetic signals, and then by applying a magnetic field to the molecules, the MRI machine can generate images of different phases of magnetization. This allows the MRI to detect changes in tissue that have different significance, such as differences between ischemic stroke and hemorrhagic stroke. MRI through MR spectroscopy may also help differentiate inflammation from stroke from tumor. Sometimes an MRI is performed with contrast, such as gadolinium. This contrast material allows better visualization of the arteries and better delineation of damaged or inflamed parts of the brain.

As is the case with allergies to contrast dye for CT, it is possible to have an allergy to the MRI contrast dye known as gadolinium. Allergy to MR contrast material is uncommon, occurring in 0.48% of patients who receive this material. Most of the reactions are minor, and serious reactions have been reported in 0.01% of patients. Of those patients who reacted to gadolinium, 12% had prior reactions to either iodine-based CT contrast or other contrast material, 20% had food and or drug allergies, and 2% had asthma. However, the remaining patients with a reaction did not have any prior reactions that would have alerted the doctors to this potential complication. Another population of patients who are considered high risk for a significant complication related to both CT and MRI contrast include those who are taking beta-blockers, such as atenolol, or those with significant cardiac history. This subgroup of patients may have a higher risk if they develop an allergic reaction because their ability to react to systemic changes may be compromised by the beta-blocker or their underlying medical condition. To help prevent reactions to these contrast agents, pretreatment with steroids and other drugs has been advocated for those patients with known allergy to contrast agents. In patients with significantly compromised kidney function it is best to avoid any contrast agent.

There are several limitations to MRI. Patients may experience claustrophobia because of the need to lie in a fairly narrow tube for upward of 45 minutes and therefore may not tolerate the procedure. For those patients there is another option, an "open MRI." Although the patient is less confined in an open MRI, this is sometimes not sufficient for patients with extreme claustrophobia. Images from open MRI may not be as detailed as a regular MRI. The use of sedatives may help minimize the anxiety during the test. Newer "high field" open MRI may eventually solve that problem. Patients receiving sedatives for the test should not drive to and from the MRI center. Another limitation is that MRI is extremely sensitive to motion. Therefore images are compromised in a patient who is unable to lie comfortably with minimal to no movement. Finally, because MRI is simply a large magnet, there is a potential for movement or heating of certain metals implanted in the body. The radiologist needs to know about any implanted metal or devices in the body, such as a defibrillator/pacemaker, before an individual can be cleared for the MRI.

PART TWO

Symptoms of Transient Ischemic Attacks and Strokes

What are the common symptoms of transient ischemic attacks and stroke?

What is neglect syndrome?

What is aphasia?

More . . .

Vertebral arteries

Two arteries in
the back of the
neck that merge
to form the basilar
artery to supply the
brainstem and the
posterior part of the
brain, including the
occipital lobes and
parts of the temporal
lobes.

Basilar artery

A major artery
supplying the back
of the brain formed
by the merger of
the two vertebral
arteries.

Carotid arteries

Two arteries in the
front of the neck
supplying most of
the blood to the
anterior part of the
brain.

Circle of Willis

Connections of
arteries inside the
brain between
arteries from the
left and right as well
as the anterior and
posterior circulation.
These connections
help maintain flow
in case one of the
arteries is blocked.

The neurological symptoms associated with transient ischemic attacks and strokes depend on the location of the diseased artery, the final location of an obstructing blood clot, or, in the case of hemorrhage, the location of the hemorrhage. Different arteries supply different parts of the brain, and different parts of the brain perform different functions. Two arteries in the back of the neck, known as the **vertebral arteries**, travel up to the base of the skull and merge to form the **basilar artery**. Branches from the vertebral and basilar arteries supply the upper part of the spinal cord and the brainstem. The brainstem contains pathways or centers for sensory, motor, balance, speech, swallowing, eye control, and vision. The brainstem is located in the "posterior fossa" of the skull (i.e., the back part of the skull) and the blood supply to that area is often referred to as the "posterior circulation." There are two arteries in the front of the neck, known as the **carotid arteries**. The common carotid arteries originate from the major vessels off the heart and then split into the external carotid artery and the internal carotid artery. The internal carotid artery supplies the anterior part of the brain or more than two thirds of the brain. The major branches of the internal carotid artery are the middle cerebral artery, the anterior cerebral artery, the ophthalmic artery, and the posterior communicating artery. Inside the brain, branches from the posterior circulation merge with branches from the anterior circulation in the **circle of Willis**. These connections between the posterior and anterior circulation allow for backup blood flow or collaterals in case one of the arteries is blocked. The circle of Willis may not be complete (i.e., lacking in one or more of the connections). Incomplete circle of Willis may impact the ability of the individual to compensate for a decrease in blood flow to parts of the brain.

Because the carotid arteries supply a large portion of the brain as well as the eyes, 75% of transient ischemia/strokes occur in those territories. The remaining transient ischemic attacks/strokes occur in the vertebral and basilar arteries. Although the symptoms of transient ischemia are transient, lasting generally less than an hour, they are not different from the permanent symptoms of stroke. A transient ischemic attack may occur in isolation without recurrence for days or weeks. Other transient ischemic attacks may reoccur several times during an hour. Both types of ischemic attacks require immediate attention because the risk of stroke after a transient ischemic attack is very high.

Because the carotid arteries supply a large portion of the brain as well as the eyes, 75% of transient ischemia/strokes occur in those territories.

Treatment of transient ischemic attacks and strokes is discussed in detail under specific conditions. As an introduction, it is important to explain some of the major treatment options. If evaluations, clinical or otherwise, point to a specific explanation for the stroke such as carotid artery disease, then surgery on the carotid artery may be necessary. The use of antiplatelet drugs (drugs that inhibit the ability of platelets to clump), such as aspirin, clopidogrel, ticlopidine (Ticlid), or Aggrenox, are helpful in a variety of conditions to prevent secondary events, such as strokes and heart attacks. **Warfarin** (Coumadin) has indirect effects on the clotting system, unrelated to platelets. Warfarin inhibits vitamin K, which is an important element in the formation of clotting factors. **Heparin** and heparin-like drugs, such as low-molecular-weight heparin, act by direct effects on the clotting cascade, but heparin can also have effects on inflammation and platelets. These drugs serve different purposes for different types of ischemic strokes.

Warfarin

Generic name for Coumadin, a blood-thinning medication that acts by inhibiting vitamin K and results in "thinning" the blood.

Heparin

Blood-thinning medications that can be given intravenously or subcutaneously.

7. What are the common symptoms of transient ischemic attacks and stroke?

Symptoms of transient ischemic attacks or stroke are variable depending on the "real estate" involved. For example, blockage of the lower branch of the middle cerebral artery in the left part of the brain causes problems in comprehending spoken and written language. Blockage of a branch of the basilar artery, affecting the brainstem, can cause double vision. However, no matter what artery or part of the brain is involved, the symptoms always start abruptly.

Symptoms of carotid artery disease (supply the front of the brain) are as follows:

- Loss of vision in one eye, partially or totally
- Numbness/tingling in face and/or hand
- Speech or language difficulties
- Weakness in left or right upper and/or lower limb

Symptoms of vertebral and basilar artery disease (supply the back part of the brain) are as follows:

- Double vision
- True vertigo, with spinning and unsteadiness
- Loss of vision, not initially perceived by the patient
- Numbness on half of the body
- Weakness or clumsiness
- Slurring of speech

I had a right hemisphere hemorrhagic stroke that damaged nearly 40% of the right side of my brain, severely impacting the left side of my body, particularly the motor skills of my limbs. Initially, I was completely paralyzed on my left side, but there were other deficits as well, especially with sensation. My whole left side felt as if it were numbed with Novocain. I had hypersensitivity to pain, temperature extremes, and, oddly, any metal object that touched my skin. Other symptoms included neglect, proprioception, spasticity, and tone. To this day, I still suffer many of these conditions although the intensity has changed.

8. What is neglect syndrome?

Neglect occurs because of damage to the right parietal part of the brain. This is a very dramatic problem, whereby the patient is unable to recognize the existence of the left side of the body or appreciate events occurring in the left visual space. Patients also do not recognize that they have developed this problem, because they do not "see" the deficit. This condition is believed to be related to damage to parts of the brain responsible for three-dimensional appreciation of the environment, including our own body parts. Depending on the size of the stroke and the extent of involvement of other nearby structures, the neglect syndrome may not be accompanied by true weakness.

However, because of profound neglect the patient is unable to move the limb or react to stimulation of the limb. Many patients with neglect do not participate in rehabilitation well, and the recovery is generally slower than other patients with pure motor strokes.

Left-side neglect syndrome, which was something I neither knew about nor understood, was my most severe and frustrating condition. While being neurologically tested in ICU, I was asked to draw the time 10:50. I drew 2:10. After two more attempts with the same results, I was asked to draw the face of a clock. I drew only the right side of the clock with the numbers 12 to 6, the left side of the clock was completely blank. Half a clock. I knew it was wrong, but I didn't know how to fix it. I couldn't read because the left side of the page was non-existent. Nothing made sense to me, but not because I couldn't see it. It was a cognitive deficit, how my brain was interpreting things. This extended to the left side of my body—nothing existed on the left side of my world. This condition has continued to plague me ten years post stroke. In fact, for the first few years, there were signs posted throughout my house, reminding me to "think left." Even now, I continue to bump into whatever might be on my left side. I also have to make a conscious effort to do the simplest activities. When walking, I must think to move my left leg forward or when climbing stairs, I must think to lift my left foot above the riser.

9. What is aphasia?

Aphasia refers to language dysfunction. In most patients the language areas are located in the left hemisphere. Language is clearly one of the more complex areas of the brain and requires input from several different sources, including higher auditory and visual information. This information is then fed to the language areas for decoding or to generate language. Although there are many different types of language dysfunction, for the sake of simplicity we can divide the language disorders into anterior versus posterior. The anterior language dysfunction is related to lesions in the frontal lobe, where the ability to generate full sentences or even words is impaired.

Because this is a language problem, even attempts at writing fail. Over time, patients may be able to communicate with single words or short sentences. Sometimes patients are able to use profanities easily but cannot say simple words. Recovery from this type of stroke is very slow. A posterior aphasia is a language dysfunction with pronounced difficulties in comprehension. The lesion is usually in the left posterior temporal part of the brain. There is often associated "word salad" where patients mix up words in a sentence or substitute words with similar sounding words. Of interest is that many patients with posterior aphasia appear to be agitated and are often brought to the emergency room with "confusion." Making the correct diagnosis can be initially difficult because the aphasia may not be obvious or as dramatic as one would expect from a stroke. Patients may be conversant but often have difficulties following commands. Furthermore, patients with damage to the posterior temporal area may have accompanying visual impairment of the right visual field. As with all aphasias, recovery is often slow and frustrating. Patients generally have difficulties following instructions or interacting with their family and medical staff. However, as with most strokes, recovery begins within a few days, and some noticeable improvements can occur over several weeks.

10. Is dizziness a sign of stroke?

Dizziness is a very common complaint. However, it is one of the least specific complaints unless it has certain characteristics. True vertigo with spinning is more concerning for a neurological problem than episodes of lightheadedness. Lightheadedness requires a workup, but generally this is not a neurological problem. Spinning-type dizziness usually originates from the inner ear balance system, the brain, or the neck. As in most neurological conditions, obtaining a good history of the symptoms is critical. The sudden onset of vertigo with nausea and vomiting, unsteadiness, and sometimes double vision and headaches is concerning for disease of the blood flow to the brainstem. The brainstem regulates some basic functions, including balance, eye movements, and sensory and motor pathways. Sometimes differentiating between vertigo originating from the inner ear and that originating from the brainstem can be difficult. A fairly common cause of vertigo is inner ear disease. Some inner ear disease causes benign positional vertigo. This condition is distinct in that the vertigo is caused by specific head and neck movements. Because the inner ear can suffer from a multitude of other conditions that cause vertigo, it may not be easy to clinically decide on the exact cause, therefore requiring imaging studies of the brain and perhaps a full evaluation of inner ear function.

11. Is blurring of vision a sign of stroke?

Not all blurry vision is associated with blood restrictions to the brain or the eyes. Sometimes differentiating among the many different reasons for blurry vision is difficult and requires input from a neurologist and an ophthalmologist. For the most part, when the visual changes are primarily those of bright, moving, and shimmering objects that evolve over few minutes and last for 20 minutes, the diagnosis is migraines, even without an associated headache. These types of visual changes are referred to as ocular migraines. These episodes may occur without a history of migraines and can start after the age of 50. Although this phenomenon involves both eyes, most patients appreciate the symptoms in one eye, making the clinical diagnosis somewhat more difficult. The typical problem related to blood flow abnormalities is the transient partial or total loss of vision in one eye. Such presentation deserves urgent evaluation. In older individuals a condition known as giant cell arteritis in which there is inflammation of the temporal artery and sometimes of the ophthalmic artery can lead to blindness if left untreated. The symptoms of giant cell arteritis include headaches, malaise, and pain in the jaw while chewing. Another condition that can lead to visual disturbance in the eye without pain is that known as anterior ischemic optic neuropathy. The cause of this condition is not entirely clear but is believed to be related to insufficient blood to the optic nerve. Because eye problems can be complicated, obtaining a baseline study of the carotid arteries or studying the blood flow through the ophthalmic artery in addition to a full neurological and ophthalmological evaluation is important to rule out problems with the eye or blood flow to the eye.

12. What is "locked-in syndrome"?

This perhaps is the cruelest type of stroke and is often misdiagnosed. Locked-in syndrome is the result of a large stroke in the pons. The pons is a major passageway for sensory and motor pathways. Blockage of the basilar artery results in this type of stroke. As a result of damage to the pons, patients are unable to move any of the limbs and lose control of horizontal eye movements. Recognizing the neurological deficits may be difficult. Neurological examination often reveals that the patient is awake and can only move the eyes vertically. The patient can comprehend conversation but cannot respond, except by blinking and with vertical eye movements. If recognized early, possible interventions with clot-busting drugs can be attempted. Generally, the morbidity and mortality of this disease is very high.

13. How often do you get headaches with stroke?

Headaches at the onset of stroke have been documented with different types of strokes. In ischemic strokes the incidence varies from 15% to 35%, whereas in intracerebral hemorrhage it occurs in as many as 40% to 60% of patients.

Headaches at the onset of stroke have been documented with different types of strokes. In ischemic strokes the incidence varies from 15% to 35%, whereas in intracerebral hemorrhage it occurs in as many as 40% to 60% of patients. In ischemic stroke headaches are more frequent in patients with posterior circulation strokes, **dissection**, or complete blockage of a major artery. The headache is usually not permanent. The location of the headache does not usually help in making a diagnosis of stroke. The sudden onset of a severe headache needs to be evaluated as soon as possible because it may be an indication of **subarachnoid hemorrhage**. Patients suffer from subarachnoid hemorrhage as a result of an **aneurysm** that burst open, allowing blood to spread in and around the brain. This is a dangerous condition that requires immediate attention.

In the days leading up to my stroke, I had a bad cold with congestion, accompanied by a headache due to the sinus pressure. Then, two hours prior to my hemorrhage, I had taken an over the-counter-cold medicine. Once my hemorrhage began, I had excruciating pain on the right side of my head. This headache was like no other I had ever experienced. I couldn't sit, stand, or lie down without doubling over in pain. It felt like a volcanic eruption in my head. I didn't know it at the time, but whenever my blood pressure pulsed, it was releasing blood into my brain.

Dissection

Separation of the layers of the arterial wall, causing narrowing and potentially resulting in stroke. This condition can occur spontaneously or with trauma.

Subarachnoid hemorrhage

Bleeding on the surface of the brain related to trauma or aneurysm.

Aneurysm

Outgrowth of an artery and rarely a vein, with a potentially weakened wall, that may bleed.

PART THREE

Types of Strokes

What is a lacunar stroke?

What is an embolic stroke?

More . . .

Several registries for stroke have been published over the years. Some of the more comprehensive registries include the Harvard Stroke Registry published in 1978, the Reese Stroke Registry published in 1983, and the Lausanne Stroke Registry published in 1988. All these registries demonstrate that the most common type of stroke is ischemic, accounting for approximately 80% of all strokes; hemorrhagic (bleeding) strokes account for 11% to 22% of all strokes. These registries further classified the subtypes of ischemic and hemorrhagic strokes (Table 1).

Table 1   Classification of stroke subtypes

Ischemic		Hemorrhagic		
Lacune	Occlusive	Embolic	SAH	ICH
13–19%	18–43%	20–31%	6–8%	10–14%

Lacunar stroke

Stroke related to the small arteries in the deep parts of the brain.

Lacunar strokes are found in the deep parts of the brain and are related to disease in the small arteries. Occlusive disease is seen in the larger vessels in the neck and near or inside the brain. Embolic strokes are caused by clots traveling from the heart or arteries to block arterial supply to parts of the brain. There are several different types of hemorrhage: intracerebral hemorrhage, which refers to bleeding inside the brain, and subarachnoid hemorrhage, which refers to bleeding around the brain caused by aneurysms or trauma and subdural and epidural hemorrhages which occur outside the brain. The latter two hemorrhages will not be discussed in this book. As mentioned earlier, approximately 30–40% of ischemic strokes occur without a definable cause. Figure 1 shows computed tomography images of the brain demonstrating the appearance of hemorrhagic stroke and ischemic stroke.

14. What is a lacunar stroke?

Lacunae or lakes refer to holes in the deep parts of the brain that are generally around 5 mm or one fifth of an inch in diameter. There are some common locations for lacunae that

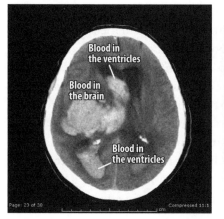 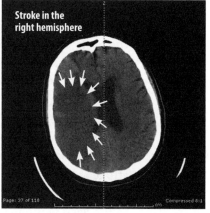

Figure 1   CT scans of the brain. On the left is a cerebral hemorrhage. On the right is an ischemic stroke.

include putamen, pons, internal capsule, and thalamus. Lacunae occur as a result of blockage of blood flow through a small artery, causing a stroke. The blockage of the artery is thought to be related to damage within the wall of the artery, resulting in thickening of the inside wall and causing an ischemic stroke or, in some cases, dilation of the outside wall, resulting in bleeding. In some pathological studies it appears that some "lacunar" strokes contain debris consistent with embolus. The extent of the stroke and ultimate effect of the stroke depend on the location and size of the embolus. As a result, a small embolus made up of cholesterol may lodge itself in the deep arteries, causing a stroke that appears like a lacuna. A thorough investigation of the source of the stroke is always warranted.

The major cause of lacunar stroke is believed to be high blood pressure, which is found in up to 75% of patients with lacunar strokes. Diabetes is another important contributor to developing lacunar disease. The major symptoms of a lacunar stroke include pure weakness or pure sensory deficits on one side of the body. Other symptoms such as double vision or speech difficulties with hand clumsiness can occur as a result of lacunar stroke in the brainstem. Because lacunar disease is a reflection of important risk factors for stroke, it is not surprising to find that many patients with this type of problem also have disease in the large arteries in the neck supplying blood to the brain. Many patients with lacunar stroke develop transient symptoms or fluctuating symptoms over several days, ultimately developing a fixed deficit. In rare cases, stuttering symptoms can occur over several weeks, with transient ischemic attack-like spells, eventually causing a stroke with fixed deficits. This latter type of presentation is difficult to diagnose as a pure lacunar stroke and may in fact be related to disease of a somewhat larger feeding artery, ultimately affecting its smallest branch in the deep white matter.

On imaging studies of the brain, especially MRI, many patients seem to have had other lacunar strokes, often asymptomatic. There are few patients who seem to have multiple lacunar infarcts in a short period of time and other patients who develop extensive amount of lacunar strokes in conjunction with diffuse or patchy changes in the white matter. This combination of changes is believed to underlie the cognitive changes, gait difficulties, and movement abnormalities seen in some patients.

Secondary prevention of lacunar strokes may be accomplished by aggressive control of risk factors. The use of aspirin or aspirin-like medications may be the only available agents for this condition. Studies using warfarin for lacunar strokes have so far not demonstrated any benefits to warfarin over aspirin. A large subgroup of the WARSS trial published in 2001 was made up of patients with lacunar strokes. The patients were randomized to receive either warfarin or aspirin and were followed for 2 years. Analysis of outcome in the two treatment groups suggest no benefit of warfarin over aspirin and that warfarin contributed to a greater risk of hemorrhage. Figure 2 shows MRIs of an isolated lacunar stroke in a typical location in a deep part of the brain as well as more diffuse "white matter disease."

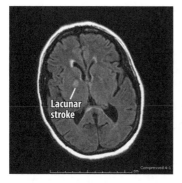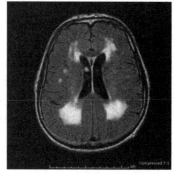

Figure 2   MRIs. On left, an isolated lacunar stroke in a typical location—a deep part of the brain. On right, more diffuse "white matter disease."

15. What is an embolic stroke?

An embolus refers to loose material that travels through the arterial system and eventually becomes stuck in a smaller artery to cause a stroke. The embolic material can be a collection of clumped platelets or platelets with red blood cells, calcium, cholesterol, bacteria, or even air. There are many causes for this problem, including irregular heart beat, such as atrial fibrillation; low cardiac output; recent myocardial infarction (heart attack); patent foramen ovale; infection on the valves (endocarditis); disease of the aortic arch; disease of large vessels in the neck; disease of arteries inside the brain (intracranial vessels); and clotting disorders. These disease processes that lead to strokes are discussed throughout this book.

In evaluating patients for a cardiac cause of strokes, physicians rely on clinical history, findings on examination such as irregular heart beat or murmurs, and findings on electrocardiogram and echocardiogram. There are two different types of echocardiograms, transthoracic and transesophageal. A transthoracic echocardiogram is the easiest cardiac ultrasound to perform. An ultrasound probe is placed on the front of the chest and images of the heart chambers are obtained. The major limitation of the transthoracic echocardiogram is that it does not adequately evaluate the entire left atrium and does not see the aortic arch. A transesophageal echocardiogram uses a probe the size of the thumb and is placed in the esophagus, which lies directly behind the heart. When the transesophageal echocardiogram is performed the physician applies numbing medication to the back of the mouth to prevent gagging and the patient is given sedating medication. Physicians can choose the appropriate type of cardiac ultrasound based on the clinical suspicion of underlying heart abnormalities.

PART FOUR

Cardiac Causes for Stroke

What is atrial fibrillation?

What is a paradoxical embolus?

What is the risk of stroke after a heart attack?

More . . .

16. What is atrial fibrillation?

Atrial fibrillation is a when the heart generates inefficient and irregular electrical impulses, resulting in abnormal contractions of the heart chambers. Sometimes this occurs in the presence of a "floppy" left atrium in which clots may form (Figure 3). These clots can then break off and cause embolic strokes. These embolic events can affect other organs in the body, including the bowels and the kidneys. It is estimated that 2.3 million individuals in the United States suffer from atrial fibrillation and that atrial fibrillation accounts for approximately 69,000 strokes per year. Seventy-five percent of patients with atrial fibrillation are between ages 65 and 85 years. Usually, atrial fibrillation is associated with other high-risk conditions such as hypertension, diabetes, and valvular disease. Patients with heart failure have high incident of atrial fibrillation. Approximately 5% of patients with atrial fibrillation suffer from stroke per year, although the risk is much higher in patients with abnormal mitral valve, the valve between the left atrium and the left ventricle. The cause of the stroke in atrial fibrillation is complex, and one fourth of strokes in patients with atrial fibrillation may not be directly related to atrial fibrillation. Treatment with warfarin is recommended for patients at high risk of embolic strokes; this issue is discussed in detail in Part 11 (see Question 85).

17. What is a paradoxical embolus?

A paradoxical embolus is embolic material that has traveled from the venous side to the arterial side, causing end-organ damage, such as a stroke. The most common source of a paradoxical embolus is the presence of a hole, known as patent foramen ovale, between the right side of the heart and the left side of the heart, allowing for a clot from the venous system to travel to the arterial system (Figure 4). However, any connection that allows venous blood to directly communicate with the arterial system via a significant passage way (i.e., fistula), as may occur in patients with pulmonary arterial–venous fistulas, can also cause a paradoxical embolus.

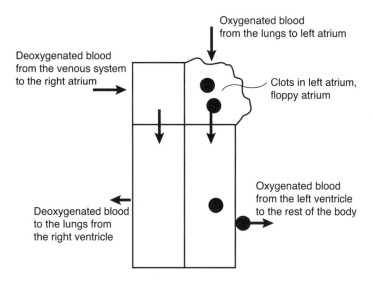

Figure 3   Circulation through the heart. Clots in left atrium, atrial fibrillation.

Patent foramen ovale is a remnant of a developmentally important connection between the right and the left sides of the heart that shunts blood away from the lungs while the fetus is still developing in the uterus. By the age of 1 year, the foramen ovale usually closes, preventing further shunting of blood from the right side to the left side via the heart. However, in approximately 25% of people the hole remains open, or patent, hence "patent foramen ovale." In young patients with stroke the prevalence of a patent foramen ovale is approximately 45%; it is therefore argued that patent foramen ovale must be an important factor that results in ischemic strokes in young individuals. Other observations regarding patent foramen ovale have been made over the years, including the possible relationship between patent foramen ovale and migraines with aura.

Some studies have suggested that the recurrence rate of stroke for patients with patent foramen ovale over 1 year is approximately 0.5%. However, the risk of recurrence is

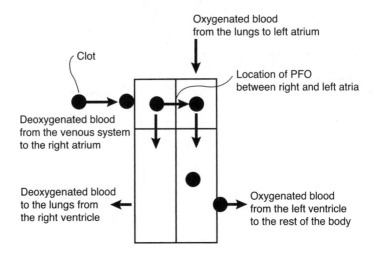

Figure 4   Circulation through the heart. Paradoxical embolus.

approximately 4% per year if the PFO is associated with an outpouching, known as an aneurysm. In young individuals with stroke but without cardiac abnormalities, the risk of stroke varies from 0% to 1%. Randomized clinical trials are attempting to address the best possible treatment for young patients with stroke and patent foramen ovale. However, these clinical trials are not enrolling patients who have patent foramen ovale associated with aneurysm, because these patients are considered to be empirically the best candidates for closure of the patent foramen ovale, due to the high risk of stroke.

The general conclusions that can be drawn from available studies are that patent foramen ovale with aneurysm poses the highest risk for recurring stroke. Closing the patent foramen ovale under those circumstances is reasonable. For all other patients, however, the recommendations await the results of the randomized clinical studies.

18. What is the risk of stroke after a heart attack?

As mentioned earlier, disease of the coronary arteries and stroke coexist, as a reflection of generalized vascular disease. However, more importantly is the risk of stroke as a direct result of the heart attack, due primarily to irregular heart beat, clots in the cardiac chambers, or immobile segments of the wall of the heart chambers that promote clot formation. Traditionally and based on clinical studies, the risk of stroke after heart attacks was estimated at 1.5% in the initial 30 days after the attack. However, because of the relatively short duration of follow-up in some studies, the incidence may be underestimated. In fact, a long-term community-based study of stroke incidence after myocardial infarction demonstrated that during a median period of 5.6 years, there was a 44-fold increase risk for stroke during the first 30 days after the heart attack. Factors that appear to increase the risk of stroke after a heart attack include advanced age, hypertension, diabetes, anterior location of the heart attack, heart failure, and atrial fibrillation. Unfortunately, prevention strategies for these types of stroke are unknown. The use of antiplatelet agents (those that prevent platelets from clumping together) such as aspirin or clopidogrel, is common after a heart attack. However, the use of warfarin has also been advocated in cases where clots can be demonstrated on the weakened wall of the heart or where a large infarct involves the anterior wall of the heart.

Disease of the coronary arteries and stroke coexist.

Cardiac Causes for Stroke

19. What is endocarditis?

Endocarditis is an infection of the heart valves. The infection can involve either the right or the left heart valves. In individuals with a history of intravenous drug abuse, the right heart valves are infected, whereas in those without a history of intravenous drug abuse, the left heart valves are involved. The heart valves are usually infected with common bacteria such as streptococci, enterococci, and *Haemophilus*. Fungus can also infect the valves, but this usually occurs in patients who are immunocompromised. In some cases the infection of the valve evolves rapidly, whereas in others the progression is more indolent. The inflammatory elements and the bacteria (vegetation) can break off; as a result, patients with left valvular endocarditis can develop signs of embolic material in the periphery such as near the nail beds. This infectious debris can infiltrate the vessel wall and cause "vasculitis," or inflammation, within the wall of the arteries. This process is widespread; it can involve any organ, including the brain. Strokes, abscesses (pockets of white blood cells and bacteria), and "mycotic" aneurysms can develop in the brain. The diagnosis of this condition can be difficult; as a result diagnostic criteria have been created to help with that process. The Duke Criteria, published in 1994, have been shown to be reliable. These criteria take into account two major factors, a positive blood culture from two separate specimens and a positive echocardiogram (ultrasound of the heart), and several minor criteria, such as predisposing heart condition, intravenous drug abuse, and fevers. Of interest, many physicians also use the erythrocyte sedimentation rate or ESR (a simple blood test) as a crude screen of inflammation in patients with stroke to guide further investigation into the possibility of endocarditis. However, an elevated ESR is not considered part of the diagnostic criteria because it is not specific enough.

Treatment of endocarditis is aimed at eradicating the bacteria with antibiotics. Endocarditis is associated with multiple secondary complications that influence recovery, including congestive heart failure, systemic embolization (widespread embolic debris), abscesses, and aneurysms. Neurological complications can occur in approximately 25% of patients with endocarditis. Vegetation on the mitral valve, one of two valves on the left side of the heart, is the source of most embolic events. The larger the vegetation, the more likely an embolic event will occur. Once a piece of the vegetation breaks off and embolizes to the brain, it can cause a stroke. Seeding of the brain with bacteria and other debris from vegetation can result in the development of abscesses, which may be difficult to treat, because the antibiotics may not reach those areas. An uncommon but serious complication of endocarditis is the development of mycotic aneurysms, which are aneurysms caused by growth of fungi or bacteria within the wall of the artery. This problem has been reported to occur in 5% of cases. A ruptured mycotic aneurysm results in a devastating outcome. Treatment is still aimed at resolving the infection, which often leads to reduction in risk of developing the secondary events. Treatment with the appropriate antibiotics even for 2 weeks significantly reduces the risk of these complications. Some mycotic aneurysms may heal with antibiotics or shrink in size, whereas other aneurysms may require monitoring or intervention.

20. Can strokes occur as a result of aortic arch disease?

The aorta is the large artery that exits the left ventricle and supplies blood to the entire body. As the aorta exits the heart it makes a turn upward and posterior before it dips down into the chest; this turn is the aortic arch. The aortic arch is exposed to significant turbulence, which over time can lead to stress injury to the wall of the artery and result in accelerating the formation of atherosclerotic disease. Atherosclerotic disease in this large artery can attract clots, and clots can then break off to cause strokes. But even without clots, atherosclerotic changes in the wall of the artery can be a significant cause of strokes either spontaneously or as a result of intervention, as may occur during cardiac catheterization and open heart surgery. An important study on this issue published in 1994 used transesophageal ultrasound of the heart to evaluate the presence and characteristics of plaque in the aortic arch in patients with a recent ischemic stroke. The study concluded that plaques equal to or larger than 4 mm (1 inch = 26 mm) had a significantly higher risk for stroke compared with smaller plaque. The larger plaque was an independent risk factor for stroke in patients over the age of 60. Some studies have suggested that large and complex plaques in the aortic arch can be found in 30% of elderly patients with stroke and may account for a significant portion of cryptogenic strokes. "Cryptogenic" strokes refer to strokes with an unknown cause and may account for 40% of all strokes.

However, if we take into consideration plaques in the aortic arch as a potential source of strokes often not appreciated by routine testing, then it is likely that more patients with so-called cryptogenic stroke can be diagnosed more appropriately. The presence of this disease in the aortic arch may be suggested by an enlarged left ventricle, which in one study was found in 90% of patients with aortic plaque and only in 30% of patients without a plaque. Because it is easier to diagnose an enlarged left ventricle by either x-ray or routine, transthoracic, cardiac ultrasound, its presence may help in guiding further testing or treatment.

The larger issue, however, is how to treat such disease once found. The larger plaque is thought to contain several different elements that can contribute to debris that result in stroke, including clots, cholesterol, inflammatory cells, and calcium. The cause of these plaques is related to the same general risk factors that lead to atherosclerotic disease, such as hypertension, smoking, diabetes, and elevated cholesterol. Treatment for aortic arch disease is unknown. Some physicians have favored warfarin, whereas others have favored antiplatelet agents (aspirin or aspirin-like drugs) in addition to risk modification and high doses of lipid-lowering drugs. There have been reports in the literature regarding surgery on the aortic arch, but this is a fairly extensive and risky surgery and is of unclear benefits. Some physicians use warfarin for a predefined period of time and then reevaluate the plaque with another transesophageal ultrasound to see whether the plaque or clot or mobile elements associated with the plaque have healed. If healing has occurred, then warfarin may be stopped. Some studies, however, suggest that this approach may give physicians a false sense of security because plaque may attract clots again and may not completely heal. Some physicians have also suggested that warfarin in aortic arch disease is inadvisable because it may lead to a condition known as "blue toe syndrome." Blue toe syndrome essentially describes the appearance of the digits due to the blockage in many small blood vessels from a shower of cholesterol emboli. This phenomenon is not unique to the use of warfarin and may occur under many circumstances when cholesterol emboli are released from the wall of the artery, abdominal aneurysm, or from under a clot that dissolved. Many physicians believe that the best treatment option is to use high-dose **statins** (a class of cholesterol-lowering drugs) in addition to antiplatelet agents (aspirin or aspirin-like drugs) and a special class of antihypertensive drugs known as "ACE inhibitors."

Statins
Class of cholesterol-lowering drugs.

21. How common are strokes from cardiac procedures?

A significant number of strokes occur while patients are hospitalized for medical or surgical reasons. Estimates for in-hospital strokes range from 6.5% to 15.0% of all strokes. Two large clusters of in-hospital strokes occur in patients with open heart surgery and cardiac catheterization. These procedures have inherit risk of stroke because of the presence of plaque in the aorta, coexisting carotid disease, or other neurovascular disease and hemodynamic changes (blood pressure changes) during surgery. Some patients suffer from neurological after-effects from these procedures. After coronary artery bypass surgery 1% to 5% of patients suffer from strokes and 30% of patients have cognitive deficits 3 months after the surgery. Even in patients who do not show neurological symptoms, coronary artery bypass graft has been shown to be associated with "silent" strokes, based on MRI studies. Small studies using two different approaches to bypass, one with the use of a cardiopulmonary bypass pump and one without a pump, demonstrated no differences in the rate of these silent infarcts or in the observed outcome at 3 months. The number of silent infarcts seems to be dependent in part on the extent of disease in the aortic arch, which can be severe in approximately 20% of patients over the age of 70.

Cardiac catheterization is done to study the coronary arteries, to evaluate heart chambers, and to treat the coronary arteries. The procedure is done by feeding a catheter through an artery in the groin, known as the femoral artery, which is then advanced through the aortic arch and then into the coronary arteries. The catheters and wires used are generally soft and flexible, but having wires and catheters pushed through the arteries may cause debris in the wall of the arteries to break off or may cause clots to form around the catheter or cause damage to the artery. Although blood-thinning medication is used during these procedures to prevent clots from forming, loose debris from dislodged material from the wall of the artery is difficult to stop using current techniques. A large study evaluated the occurrence of strokes during 20,924 cardiac catheterization procedures. The rate of clinically evident strokes was 0.11%. Some patients suffer from multiple strokes and some patients appear to suffer from a shower of cholesterol emboli involving multiple organs. The strokes resulted in the death of 32%, and many patients suffered from significant disability as a result of the stroke. This and other studies also demonstrated that stroke risk from the procedure is highest in those with severe coronary artery disease, perhaps reflecting the need to perform more complicated and longer procedures. Other studies have also demonstrated a relationship between disease in the aortic arch and the risk of stroke. As with any complex procedure, the risks and the benefits need to be discussed with the medical team whenever possible. Cardiac catheterization, however, may be the only available test to help diagnose a heart condition. Advances in imaging using MRI and CT may provide an alternative in the future in some cases.

PART FIVE

Strokes From the Carotid and Vertebral Arteries

How do you diagnose disease in the carotid and vertebral arteries?

How do you treat symptomatic carotid disease?

Should you treat asymptomatic carotid narrowing?

More . . .

There are two major causes of disease in the carotid and vertebral arteries, atherosclerotic disease and dissection. Atherosclerotic disease is the most common cause of disease in the carotid and vertebral arteries. Atherosclerosis can affect any artery in the body and is the result of "fatty" deposits, local inflammation, calcium, and reorganization of a segment of the artery. Common locations for atherosclerotic changes include the origin of the internal carotid artery and the origin of the vertebral artery and near the base of the skull. It has been estimated that some form of atherosclerotic disease in the carotid arteries exists in 30% of patients over the age of 60. Although this is a relatively common problem, luckily not all patients with carotid narrowing suffer from strokes.

22. How do you diagnose disease in the carotid and vertebral arteries?

The carotid artery is the major artery that supplies blood to a large part of the brain. Disease in the carotid artery usually occurs at its origin and at another area near the base of the skull. Although your doctor can listen to the neck for turbulence of flow, this by no means is either a sensitive or specific test. The easiest test to evaluate the carotid artery is an ultrasound. The ultrasound can be limited technically by the machine or the technician performing the test. The ultrasound can only see and measure flow through a small portion of the carotid system, below the angle of the jaw. The carotid extends for an additional 2 to 3 inches above the angle of the jaw and then turns into the skull, traveling up toward the brain. Because most of the disease in the carotid artery is at the origin of the internal carotid, near the angle of the jaw, carotid ultrasounds detect most carotid atherosclerotic disease. However, carotid ultrasound is only able to give us an idea of the degree of narrowing and is not an exact measurement. For example, the degree of narrowing for a given artery may be reported as 50% to 70%. As a result of these limitations, other tests are often needed to help estimate the degree of narrowing and to look at the whole extent of the carotid artery as well as other arteries.

Several tests are helpful to estimate the degree of narrowing and to look at the whole extent of the carotid artery, such as **magnetic resonance angiography (MRA), computed tomography angiography (CTA),** and the traditional angiography or digital subtraction angiography. All these tests have advantages and limitations.

The MRA can be obtained as part of an MRI, therefore obtaining images of the brain and arteries. It is best to do the MRA with gadolinium, a contrast material, to allow for better delineation of the arteries especially in tortuous segments. Many patients are claustrophobic and therefore cannot tolerate the MRI/MRA. Also, a very small number of patients are allergic to the contrast material. Patients with allergies to contrast material may receive a combination of prednisone (steroid) and diphenhydramine hydrochloride (Benadryl) before the injection of the contrast. Patients with compromised kidney function should not receive the contrast material. Another disadvantage to MRI/MRA is that the test is very sensitive to movement; therefore, a patient who cannot lie comfortably in the machine and stay for the required time of approximately 40 minutes cannot have the test. Furthermore, the MRA only provides an estimate of the extent of narrowing. Figure 5 is an MRA that shows the major arteries feeding the brain. Note differences between the narrowed left internal carotid artery and the normal right internal carotid artery.

The CTA is another noninvasive test for the arteries. This test requires the infusion of contrast. The acquisition of the images is much faster than MRA, and the images of the vessels are detailed. The CTA provides additional information not obtainable from MRA, such as the amount of calcium in the vessels, and also allows a more precise measurement of the degree of narrowing. In some areas, near the skull base, narrowing of the carotid may be difficult to differentiate from background calcification in the vessel or bone. The major disadvantage of the CTA is the amount of contrast required

Magnetic resonance angiography (MRA)

Uses MRI technology to look at arteries and veins.

Computed tomography angiography (CTA)

Noninvasive test that uses a CT with intravenous injection of dye to visualize the arteries and veins in the body.

Strokes From the Carotid and Vertebral Arteries

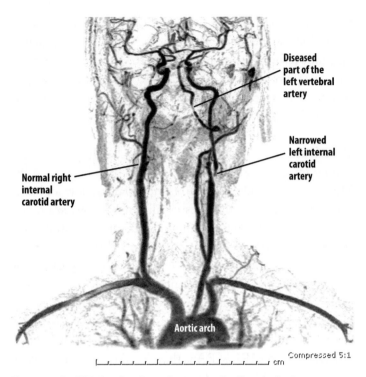

Diseased
part of the
left vertebral
artery

Narrowed
left internal
carotid
artery

Normal right
internal
carotid artery

Aortic arch

Compressed 5:1

Figure 5   An MRA showing the major arteries feeding the brain.

and possible adverse reaction in patients with poor kidney function and those taking certain medications for diabetes. Many more people have allergy to the CT contrast, but again the use of prednisone and Benadryl before the test can help prevent a significant reaction. Figure 6 shows a CTA with narrowing of the internal carotid artery.

Traditional angiography or digital subtraction angiography is an invasive test requiring the introduction of a catheter through a major artery in the groin, the femoral artery. The catheter is then advanced to the base of the major vessels in the neck where injections of contrast are made. X-ray images are then taken at different phases of the contrast injections. Traditional angiography is considered the "gold standard." However, because this is an invasive test, more complications

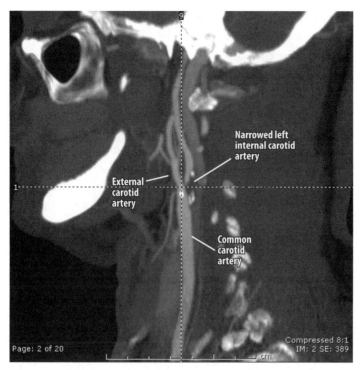

Figure 6   A CTA showing hardening of the internal carotid artery.

are reported. The complications include stroke, damage to the artery, bleeding, and reaction to the contrast material. This test is done only if all other noninvasive tests are inconclusive. MRA and CTA have evolved significantly over the past few years and likely will replace traditional angiogram.

23. How do you treat symptomatic carotid disease?

Carotid artery narrowing exists in many people without causing any symptoms. A few patients become symptomatic with transient ischemic attacks or strokes. This is often how patients present to the hospital, and some will undergo surgery to help correct the narrowing and clear the atherosclerotic debris. The timing of the surgery has been debated in the surgical literature and surgical practice is variable. In patients with a "large" stroke, many surgeons prefer to wait for few weeks before operating because of the possibility of transforming the stroke into a bleed due to opening of the narrowed artery and causing high-pressure perfusion ("flooding") of damaged brain.

The benefit of carotid surgery in patients with a recent transient ischemia or stroke has been studied extensively over the years. The NASCET study, published in 1991, randomized 659 patients to either surgery or best medical treatment. At 2 years the risk of stroke on the symptomatic side was 26% for the medical group and 9% for the surgical group. The largest risk of stroke in the surgical group was seen in the initial 30 days after the surgery at almost 6%, whereas in the medical group the risk of stroke in the initial 30 days after enrollment in the study was 3.3%. Therefore this study demonstrated that surgery was superior to medical treatment but that surgery had an upfront risk. The surgery also appeared to provide durable benefit, with steady reduction of the risk of stroke from the time of randomization until 24 months and then stabilization of this benefit. Although this study clearly demonstrated benefit to surgery, some physicians have questioned the applicability of the results to "real" patients, that is, typical patients with multiple medical problems who otherwise would have been excluded from enrollment in the NASCET study. A review of carotid surgery at the Cleveland Clinic revealed that high-risk patients had a significantly higher rate of complications from surgery. Patients who were considered high risk included those with congestive heart failure, a history of heart disease, a history of renal insufficiency and those with active lung disease. In high-risk patients the risk of stroke was 3.3%, whereas in low-risk patients the risk of stroke was 1.7%. The risk of death in the high-risk group was 4.4%, whereas the risk of death in the low-risk group was 0.3%. Complications can arise from either the anesthesia or surgery. In an attempt to minimize the risk of anesthesia in select patients, some surgeons operate on the carotid artery under local anesthesia and with sedation. As is the case with any medical

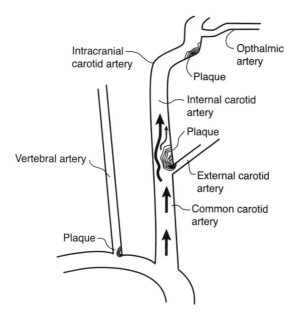

Figure 7   Carotid and vertebral artery atherosclerosis.

procedure, it is important to seek out surgeons and medical centers with extensive experience in carotid revascularization. Figure 7 shows typical location of atherosclerotic narrowing of the carotid and vertebral arteries.

Complications from carotid surgery include

- stroke
- bleeding at the site of surgery
- nerve injury, with residual hoarseness of voice
- infection
- death

24. Should you treat asymptomatic carotid narrowing?

Asymptomatic carotid narrowing is more common than symptomatic disease. This problem is often found incidentally during general physical examination when turbulent flow, a bruit, in the carotid is heard via stethoscope. The physician then usually orders a carotid ultrasound, which may reveal narrowing in the internal carotid artery. If the patient has had no symptoms to suggest transient ischemic attacks or stroke, then the carotid artery is considered asymptomatic. However, if a CT or MRI is done and an incidental stroke is found in the appropriate territory and without other explanation, some neurologists then consider the carotid artery as symptomatic. In 1995 the Asymptomatic Carotid Atherosclerosis Study (ACAS) addressed the issue of risks and benefits of surgery in patients without symptoms. In this study, 1,662 patients with 60% or greater narrowing were randomized to either surgery or best medical treatment. At 5 years the risk of stroke or death in the surgical group was 5.1% and in the medical group was 11.0%. Most of the benefit was noted in patients who had high-grade narrowing, whereas women had a higher rate of complications from the surgery. The benefit of the surgery was not immediately realized, however, with most benefit seen 36 months after the surgery. Although the evidence suggests a reduction of risk of stroke from 2% per year to 1% per year, the overall risks of the surgery and the delayed benefit of the surgery as well as other coexisting medical issues need to be considered before surgery is done. Some patients with moderate narrowing may be best watched with maximization of medical treatment and reduction of risk factors. Table 2 summarizes the risk of stroke, MI (myocardial infarction heart attack), and death in patients with asymptomatic carotid artery narrowing.

An important criticism of this study is that it followed patients for only an average of 2.7 years, but the risk was calculated over 5 years using accepted statistical methods. Therefore it is argued that the short-term follow-up in the ACAS could not adequately determine the contribution of other vascular or nonvascular problems that could influence long-term morbidity and mortality and therefore eliminating the benefits of carotid surgery in asymptomatic patients.

Table 2   A Summary of Risk

Stroke risk by degree of carotid stenosis	Risk at 10 years	Risk at 15 years
Less than 50%	5.7%	8.7%
50–99%	9.3%	16.6%
MI and death	10.1%	24.0%

In asymptomatic patients the decision to have the surgery needs to be discussed with the surgeon, the primary care physician, and, when necessary, a neurologist with expertise in vascular neurology. If you decide to proceed with surgery, you should seek out a surgeon with significant experience in carotid surgery.

Another important situation is the presence of asymptomatic carotid narrowing on the opposite side of a symptomatic carotid artery. Under those circumstances once the symptomatic carotid is addressed, the asymptomatic carotid narrowing should be monitored with ultrasound and by symptoms. Although some studies in the past suggested no benefits to monitoring with ultrasound, more recent studies published in 2007 provide important observations regarding progression of disease in asymptomatic carotid arteries and the yield of monitoring with ultrasound. In one study, over a period of 4 years, approximately 25% of patients progressed to a higher grade of narrowing. The patients with a mild amount of narrowing progressed over a longer period of time than the ones with moderate amount of narrowing. In few cases, the narrowing jumped from mild to severe. Over this period of observation, approximately 3% developed neurological symptoms, either a stroke or transient ischemic attack. However, most of these events occurred in patients who progressed from moderate to severe narrowing. This study illustrates that a significant number of patients will progress and that there is also significant unpredictability to this progression. For example, it is not clear why some

Strokes From the Carotid and Vertebral Arteries

patients progress and others do not. It is also not clear why some progression is rapid and other progression is slow and remains asymptomatic. The culmination of evidence suggests that monitoring in patients with asymptomatic stenosis using ultrasound is reasonable and that performing the monitoring every 6 months to a year may be beneficial in detecting progression. This monitoring is likely to benefit patients who are considered at high risk, such as those who have had surgery on the opposite carotid, those with coronary and peripheral vascular disease, and those with uncontrolled risk factors.

Finally, in the presence of asymptomatic completely blocked carotid artery on one side and a narrowed asymptomatic carotid artery on the opposite side, the risk of surgery on the asymptomatic side is considered high. Under those circumstances, maximizing management of risk factors is critical and may lead to stabilization of the disease.

Balloon angioplasty and stenting has evolved over the years and now is done with more flexible stents as well as with a "distal protection device."

Stent

Tubular metallic mesh that is inserted inside of a narrowed artery after the artery undergoes dilation with a balloon to maintain patency.

25. What if I do not qualify for surgery?

Many patients may be considered poor candidates for surgery because of either coexisting medical conditions or narrowing of an artery that was previously operated on. Balloon angioplasty and stenting has evolved over the years and now is done with more flexible **stents** as well as with a "distal protection device." Stents are made up of tubular wires that can expand. The use of stents decreases the risk of the vessel renarrowing. The distal protection devise is equivalent to an umbrella that is deployed just before the angioplasty is done and before the stent is placed. This "umbrella" catches debris that may form or break off during the procedure.

Experience with stenting over the years has demonstrated its utility in treating some patients with carotid narrowing. The cumulative experience of 36 centers worldwide was reviewed and published in 2000. The data demonstrated that the risk of stroke at 30 days after the procedure was 4.2% and the renarrowing rate was 3.5%. These findings suggested that the procedure was viable. The results of a randomized study were published in 2004. In this study 334 patients were randomized to either stenting or surgery. Only 30% of patients were symptomatic at the time of enrollment in the study. At 1 year the study showed that 20 of 167 patients in the stent group had either died or had a stroke, whereas in the surgery group 32 of 167 had these complications, or 12% complications in the stent group versus 20% in the surgery group. This study also noted that in the initial 30 days after the procedure nearly 5% of patients in the stent group and nearly 10% in the surgical group had died, had a stroke, or suffered a heart attack. This study is by no means a definitive study on the risk and benefits of stenting versus surgery. A careful look at the data demonstrates that in symptomatic patients the outcome was the same between the two groups. In the asymptomatic group, the majority of patients in this study, the 1-year outcome favored the stent. There have been many criticisms of this study including the inclusion of asymptomatic patients, whom if left without any intervention would have faired better. Furthermore, having a third group that was treated medically could have helped improve interpretation of the results (i.e., what if medical treatment alone, especially in the asymptomatic patients, was more effective than stent or surgery?). Finally, 20% of patients enrolled in this study were over the age of 80, and this is considered a fairly high-risk group for vascular interventions. A recent study was stopped early because it demonstrated a significantly higher risk of complications from stents in patients over the age of 80.

It is important to look at clinical studies with a critical eye to avoid major misrepresentation of the data. For example, it is not unusual to tell patients that surgery will cut the risk of stroke from asymptomatic carotid narrowing by 50%. Although this is technically correct based on the ACAS data discussed above, one has to remember that the risk of stroke is reduced from 2% per year to 1% per year. These are relatively small reductions in the risk of stroke. Although stents are an attractive alternative to a major operation, the techniques are still not perfected and additional data need to be collected to justify choosing stenting over surgery. To help you reach the best possible decision, it is best to consult with physicians who work as part of a multidisciplinary team that includes surgeons, neurologists, and experts in interventional procedures.

26. What if the carotid artery is completely blocked?

This is a difficult problem because there is no intervention currently that can unblock the artery. It is clear, however, that with a blocked carotid artery patients can suffer from strokes. The strokes are likely related to flow abnormalities instead of clot formation. One study that followed 104 patients, some with symptomatic and some with asymptomatic carotid occlusion, showed that at the end of 24 months, the risk of stroke was as high as 32%. The highest risk was found in patients with no "collateral" flow. The presence of a combination of collaterals is better than one collateral or no collaterals. Collaterals are considered "backup" connections among arteries on the inside and outside of the brain. Few neurologists have advocated the use of blood-thinning medication, such as heparin and warfarin, for a short period of time to prevent the possibility of new clots from forming and breaking off at either ends of the blocked artery. Others advocate the use of aspirin alone. This area has never been studied, and neurologists and vascular surgeons who treat patients with carotid artery disease do not agree on one specific treatment for this problem. Some argue that the major cause of stroke in patients with an occluded (blocked) carotid artery is related to flow abnormalities and not to clot. Patients who develop symptoms and who have evidence of poor collaterals or evidence of compromised flow should be considered for interventions. Some patients could benefit from a bypass of the blocked internal carotid artery. The bypass is from one of the arteries outside the brain to another artery inside the head, therefore bypassing the blocked carotid artery. Although a study of the benefits of bypass in the past did not demonstrate any benefit, that study was fraught with unfortunate poor design and patient selection; a new study is currently enrolling patients.

27. What if the narrowing of the artery is not accessible by surgery?

Most symptomatic narrowing of the carotid artery occurs at its split located near the angle of the jaw, making it easily accessible by surgery. But symptomatic narrowing of the carotid artery higher up at the skull base can occur in 10% of patients. Narrowing in the higher segments of the internal carotid artery is not reachable by open surgery. Balloon angioplasty may be the only option if intervention is necessary. Angioplasty is done via a catheter introduced in a groin artery and fed all the way to the carotid artery in the neck where the balloon is dilated, usually for multiple brief periods; a stent may be placed in the artery to keep it open. The risks to these procedures that must be considered before intervention are stroke, occlusion, dissection, and bleeding.

The WASID (Warfarin vs. Aspirin for Symptomatic Intracranial Stenosis) study published in 2001 assessed the benefits of treatment with aspirin versus warfarin to help prevent stroke from this condition. The study demonstrated no difference in outcome between those who were treated with aspirin and those who received warfarin, with overall stroke rates at approximately 17% over 2 years in either treatment group in patients with any type of intracranial disease. Critics of this study have argued that the level of anticoagulation with warfarin was suboptimal; therefore if the blood-thinning levels of warfarin were maintained at better therapeutic levels, then the warfarin group may have had better outcome. Although this criticism is valid to some extent, the WASID trial clearly demonstrated the difficulties in maintaining a therapeutic level of anticoagulation. Even in the setting of highly regimented clinical trial protocols, approximately 16% of patients had daily subtherapeutic levels of the **international**

Most symptomatic narrowing of the carotid artery occurs at its split located near the angle of the jaw, making it easily accessible by surgery.

Strokes From the Carotid and Vertebral Arteries

International normalization ratio (INR)

Blood test done to evaluate the effects of blood thinning of warfarin. The higher the INR, the "thinner" the blood. An INR of 1.0 is normal, meaning no effect of warfarin.

normalized ratio (INR); (measures the blood-thinning level of warfarin). Therefore at this time the recommendations for treating narrowing of arteries near the skull base or even in the brain are unknown. Maximizing medical therapy with antiplatelet drugs, statins, and blood pressure control is the best option we have. In patients who are symptomatic despite best medical treatment, perhaps more invasive interventions can be justified.

28. Can medication be a substitute for surgery in treating carotid disease?

Disease at the origin of the carotid artery, once symptomatic, needs to be addressed as quickly as possible to prevent future strokes. As discussed earlier, in patients with symtomatic carotid disease demonstrated that surgery is more effective than best medical treatment (see page 38 for discussion regarding the clinical trial known as NACET). However, as with any surgical or nonsurgical intervention, the risks and benefits of any intervention need to be weighted before a decision is made regarding the most appropriate treatment. It is also important to remember that the results of clinical trials do not always apply to individual patients. Although clearly surgery is more beneficial than best medical treatment in patients with symptomatic 70% or greater narrowing, the NASCET trial also provided us with information on the behavior of carotid disease. For example, at 1 year in the medical group the risk of stroke from symptomatic carotid disease decreases by half after initial presentation with transient ischemia or stroke. Although this may not be entirely comforting to a patient with concerns about having a stroke, it is helpful to understand that medical intervention and the nature of atherosclerotic disease is amenable to medical treatment. Some drugs that may prove to be extremely helpful and underused in the NASCET trial are the statins. Statin therapy for the treatment of cholesterol is discussed extensively in a different part of this book (Part 14, see Question 93). The data that we have now regarding appropriate cholesterol levels and use of statin therapy were not available when NASCET was enrolling patients and when it was published in 1995. A glimpse at the potential benefits of aggressive use of statins in atherosclerotic disease comes from the AVERT trial (Atorvastatin Versus Revascularization Treatments), which compared the benefit of aggressive lowering of cholesterol versus angioplasty in patients with stable coronary artery disease. This trial showed that patients in the atorvastatin group had an overall reduction of coronary event by 36% compared with those who underwent angioplasty. Over 10 studies have measured the benefit of lowering low-density lipoprotein (LDL; "bad") cholesterol on the thickness of the wall of the carotid artery, which is a marker of atherosclerotic disease. These studies have demonstrated a significant regression of disease with use of statins. Therefore the converging evidence suggests that aggressive lowering of LDL cholesterol and the use of statin therapy in patients with vascular disease can significantly help prevent coronary events and can help in healing atherosclerotic changes in the carotid arteries. The benefit of this treatment, however, is realized over time (i.e., several months), too long for patients with unstable vascular condition.

29. What is a dissection?

The arteries have three layers called the intima, the media, and the adventitia. In a dissection, blood seeps in behind one or two of these layers. The pressure from the constant pulsation pushes the blood further into and higher through the wall, separating the layers. This then can result in blocking the artery completely. Even if the artery does not completely close, the inside of the artery becomes irregular and can attract clots that can break off and cause a stroke. Most of the dissections involve the intima and the media and less often the adventitia. Tortuous or coiled segments of the arteries may be more susceptible to aneurysm formation. Dissection leads to ischemia (i.e., local absence of blood supply from obstruction of an artery) from clot fragments. Dissection can occur in any vessel, but some studies have suggested that there are more dissections of the vertebral artery than the carotid artery. Dissection of the internal carotid artery occurs an inch or more above the split, implying the existence of a "vulnerable" or weak area. The dissection can extend toward the head, but stops at the base of the skull and generally does not extend into the intracranial portion of the carotid. The most concerning complication from dissection is a stroke. A major stroke occurs in 20% to 30% of patients. Studies with special ultrasound, called transcranial ultrasound, have demonstrated that most strokes in dissection occur as a result of small emboli (i.e., blood clot fragments). In a small number of patients the strokes appear to be the result of decrease in the blood flow to border zone areas (i.e., areas that are marginally perfused by an artery).

Many patients with dissections present with pain and head-ache on the side of the dissection. The headache may be mild or severe but only lasts for a few days. Many patients may present with stroke as the first indication of a dissection. Under rare circumstances a dissection can present as a subarachnoid hemorrhage. Subarachnoid hemorrhage from a dissection usually occurs as a result of dissection of the vertebral artery. Figure 8 is an illustration of the changes seen in dissection.

30. What causes a dissection?

A dissection is believed to be caused by an underlying abnormality in the artery in areas where different parts of the artery are joined during early stages of development. Trauma as a major cause of dissection is well recognized. However, causes of spontaneous dissections and those caused by trivial trauma may have other more systemic reasons as the cause. Conditions such as fibromuscular dysplasia and disorders of connective tissue, including Ehlers-Danlos syndrome, pseudoxanthoma elasticum, and Marfan's syndrome, have all been associated with dissections. Many of the connective tissue diseases have familial tendencies. Therefore investigations of other unaffected family members may be warranted, especially when there is a concern about aneurysms.

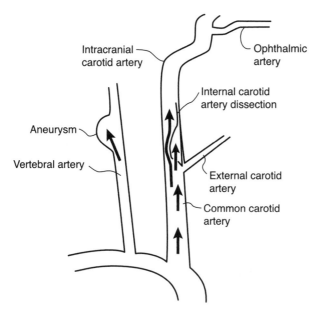

Intracranial carotid artery

Ophthalmic artery

Internal carotid artery dissection

Aneurysm

Vertebral artery

External carotid artery

Common carotid artery

Figure 8   Carotid and Vertebral artery dissections

31. What is fibromuscular dysplasia?

This is a condition that affects arteries as a result of disruption of the elastic layer in small- and medium-sized arteries. In this condition the middle layer of the artery is disrupted, resulting in weakening of the wall of the artery and the creation of loops and folds, "cork-screw"–like abnormalities. The arteries supplying the brain and those inside the brain are involved in 30% of the cases. Most of the individuals affected are females. Some patients may have aneurysms associated with this condition, with estimates of cerebral aneurysms found in 7% to 24% of patients. This condition can result in blockage, dissection, or aneurysm. In approximately 60% to 85% of cases the disorder can affect more than one artery. The carotid arteries are involved in up to 95% of the cases, and the vertebral arteries are involved in up to 43% of cases. Treatment for this condition is unknown and patients are managed in similar fashion to other patients with stroke.

32. How do you treat dissections?

There has never been a study to evaluate the benefits of different treatment options. However, nonrandomized studies (i.e., treatment at the discretion of the physician) have been published. These studies suggest that the highest risk of stroke after a dissection is in the initial 2 weeks and that the highest risk for stroke is in those with a highly narrowed artery or blocked artery. Some studies have also suggested that in spite of the use of any of the available blood-thinning medications, like warfarin, or antiplatelet drugs, like aspirin, some patients still suffer a stroke after the initial event. Other studies have demonstrated marginal benefit to warfarin over aspirin in preventing subsequent strokes. The rate of recurring stroke is not known, but some studies suggested a rate of 0.6% of subsequent stroke to more than 12% in the first year after a dissection. Because it is not known what is likely to help reduce the risk of stroke from dissection, most physicians make their own decisions regarding treatment. Some physicians initiate treatment with heparin and warfarin (blood-thinning agents), whereas others use aspirin or aspirin-like medications (drugs that inhibit the ability of platelets to clump). In the appropriate patient it is reasonable to use heparin initially and convert to warfarin, until follow-up studies demonstrate improvement or resolution of the dissection. Other interventions have been tried in some patients to include placing a stent in the artery. This intervention has also not been studied systematically, but case reports suggest that in some cases the intervention may help open the artery. Many neurologists and interventionalists do not agree on the logic behind placing a stent in the artery. Placing a stent in an artery that has a fragile wall may induce worsening of the dissection. Furthermore, aggressive dilatation of the artery could potentially lead to pushing of the clot farther up into the wall of the artery, leading to expansion of the dissection.

Approximately 85% of narrowed arteries, 50% of occluded arteries, and 43% of dissected aneurysms improve or return to normal. Healing generally occurs in the first 3 months, and vessels that do not heal by 6 months are unlikely to heal. Follow-up studies of the arteries over this period of time help to determine when it is appropriate to discontinue treatment.

33. What is a dissecting aneurysm?

This refers to the development of aneurysm (pseudoaneurysm) after a dissection. The frequency of this condition is unknown but may be as high as 50%. Aneurysms in the carotid artery after a dissection could be asymptomatic, but on occasion the pseudoaneurysm may compress nearby nerves, causing hoarseness of voice and/or swallowing difficulties. Because pseudoaneurysms of the carotid artery occur outside the brain and are surrounded by the soft tissue, bleeding may be less concerning. Pseudoaneurysm of the vertebral artery appears to be more dangerous because dissections of the vertebral artery often occur inside the skull. Although many pseudoaneurysms can heal, bleeding pseudoaneurysm can cause severe neurological deficits or death. Treatment of pseudoaneurysm include placing coils in the aneurysm, but the fragility of these pseudoaneurysms makes any mechanical disruption of the aneurysm very dangerous; as a result, occluding the feeding vessel may be necessary.

34. Can dissections reoccur?

A study from the Mayo Clinic of 200 patients with cervical arterial dissections followed for over 7 years suggested that the recurrence rate was 2% in the first month and 1% yearly thereafter. The cumulative risk of recurrent dissection over 10 years was 12%. All recurrent dissections occurred in arteries not involved by the initial dissection (other cervical arteries in 87% and renal arteries in 13%). Family history of dissection was the only predictor of recurrence. Other studies showed that recurrence was at 1% per year, occurred only at the site of the initial dissection, and correlated with the presence of fibromuscular dysplasia or Ehlers-Danlos syndrome; these conditions affect the elastic layer of the arteries.

PART SIX

Clotting Abnormalities as a Cause for Strokes

What are the common clotting disorders?

How does an abnormality in clotting factors
increase the risk for stroke?

How do you test for clotting disorders?

More . . .

Generally, clotting problems lead to clots in veins, not arteries. Luckily, it is quite uncommon for veins in the brain to clot and cause strokes. Some individuals have inherited clotting disorders that when combined with other prothrombotic (clot forming) conditions they may develop a stroke. A good example is in those patients who develop clots in a major leg vein who later have a stroke as a result of a hole in the heart, known as patent foramen ovale, or, in those patients who have a "mild" clotting disorder but develop more extensive clotting problems when placed on oral contraceptives with high estrogen content. The double hit of having a tendency to form clots combined with an additional element that causes clots can lead to serious problems.

35. What are the common clotting disorders?

Clotting disorders as a cause for stroke are more likely to become a concern when the patient is young and other traditional causes of strokes have been ruled out. Some conditions are clearly inherited, whereas other clotting disorders are acquired. A general screen for clotting can be done with simple blood tests. Clotting conditions are generally the result of a change in certain clotting proteins, which are part of the normal clotting cascade. However, other clotting conditions are triggered by other proteins that are not part of the clotting cascade. The most important proteins in that category are the antiphospholipid antibodies. These antibodies inhibit two critical proteins in the clotting cascade, protein C and protein S, and also activate the platelets. An aggressive, yet rare, form of a disease with antiphospholipid antibodies is known as Sneddon's syndrome. In this condition patients suffer from multiple episodes of venous clots, strokes and transient ischemic attacks, and even hemorrhages. It is estimated that approximately 3% to 50% of patients with Sneddon's syndrome will suffer from cerebrovascular events. But there is a spectrum of antiphospholipid disorders, including a condition that primarily affects the brain, known as Hughes syndrome. Neurological symptoms of antiphospholipid antibody syndromes include psychosis, nerve damage, Parkinson-like symptoms, multiple sclerosis–like presentation, dementia, seizures, and headaches. What causes this disorder is not fully understood, but in part a cause is inflammation of the blood vessel wall, eventually leading to formation of scar tissue followed by narrowing of the small vessels. Few patients eventually develop lupus. The diagnosis of Sneddon's syndrome can be difficult because some patients may not be positive for antiphospholipid antibodies but may exhibit skin changes with spiderweb-like discoloration, otherwise known as livedo reticularis, and vascular complications. The rate of antiphospholipid positive antibodies varies from 39% to 86% depending on the antibody test. Not all patients develop skin changes, around 40%, and skin biopsy often fails to demonstrate changes that have been reported to occur in some patients. The best treatment for symptomatic patients with the antiphospholipid antibody syndrome is unknown. Opinion papers and retrospective reviews have in some cases suggested benefits to steroids and other immunosuppressive drugs in addition to antithrombotic medications, such as aspirin or even warfarin in combination with aspirin. However, a recent randomized study comparing patients with and without antiphospholipid antibodies and strokes (APASS, 2004) demonstrated no differences in recurring strokes between patients with and without antiphospholipid antibodies or between patients who were treated with warfarin versus those treated with aspirin. Therefore at this time the presence or absence of antiphospholipid antibodies may be a reflection of autoimmune disorder that can potentially influence clotting. But the relevance of this condition to stroke is unknown. The best approach to the management of this condition is to consult a team that includes a hematologist, rheumatologist, and stroke neurologist.

Another controversial condition associated with increased risk for ischemic strokes is elevated homocysteine. The relationship between increased homocysteine and strokes is not as clear-cut as one would hope, because correcting homocysteine levels is relatively simple but does not necessarily help reverse the clotting risk. Prothrombin, a protein, as well as other factors that are important in promoting clot formation, have been found to be elevated in patients with high levels of homocysteine. Deficiencies in vitamin B_{12} and folic acid levels can cause elevated homocysteine. A genetic condition called methylenetetrahydrofolate reductase results in elevated homocysteine levels and is fairly prevalent in young patients with coronary artery disease. Treatment with folate, vitamin B_6, and/or vitamin B_{12} reduces homocysteine levels within a few weeks, but there is no evidence that such treatment decreases the risk of clotting.

36. How does an abnormality in clotting factors increase the risk for stroke?

The clotting pathways and triggers for clotting are complicated biochemical reactions that constantly balance the need to clot versus the need to prevent excessive clotting. The clotting system inside the body responds to vascular injury similar to responding to a cut on the skin. The clotting system does not differentiate between an injury on the outside and an injury on the inside of the body. The major goal is to prevent excessive loss of blood. However, the clotting system can be fooled into forming clots by certain changes in the body such as inflammation, certain medications, shearing injury to platelets going through an irregular artery, and injuries to the wall of the artery from plaques and dissections.

The clotting system is too complicated to discuss here, but the anticlotting cascade involves fewer factors and is relatively easier to appreciate. This starts by combining two proteins, thrombin and thrombomodulin, which in turn activate protein C. The activation of protein C is helped by protein S. Once activated, protein C then can inactivate two factors involved in clotting, Va and VIIIa. Increased clotting can occur as a result of mutations or changes in the level of these factors, therefore changing the balance in favor of clotting. Because of this interplay between the normal physiological response to injury and the sensitive balance between clotting and anticlotting, minor changes in the clotting system and minor vascular injury that otherwise may have been harmless can combine to cause significant clot formation, triggering an exaggerated response.

37. How do you test for clotting disorders?

There is an extensive list of blood tests that can be done to screen for clotting disorders:

- Protein C and protein S
- Antithrombin III
- Factor V Leiden
- Anticardiolipin antibodies
- Lupus anticoagulant
- Factor VIII
- Fibrinogen
- Prothrombin gene mutation (G20210A)
- D-dimer
- Platelet counts
- Hematocrit
- Prothrombin time/partial thromboplastin time
- Fasting homocysteine

However, some of the results can be equivocal, meaning that some of these can show borderline abnormalities and may not be significant on their own. Therefore input from specialists may be needed before a final determination is made regarding relevance of the findings and treatment approach. Furthermore, not all available clotting tests need to be done. Again, which tests should be done can be determined by your doctors.

38. What is the treatment for clotting abnormalities?

There are no guidelines for the treatment of asymptomatic clotting abnormalities. However, once symptoms occur, such as a stroke, there is a significant impetus to treat with warfarin (Coumadin). Although the rationale exists for using warfarin, there are no studies to support such practice. A recent clinical study addressing the use of warfarin versus aspirin in patients with the antiphospholipid syndrome found no difference between the two treatment groups. Under these circumstances, the best treatment is that based on input from multiple specialists that can assess the risk and the benefits in each case.

39. Can cancer cause a stroke?

There are many different types of cancers that have an influence on the clotting cascade that can lead to strokes (Table 3). Many patients may present for the first time with a stroke without knowing they have an underlying malignancy, whereas other patients already have advanced cancer and then present with a stroke. Although in some cases there is a direct relationship between the cancer and the stroke, in other cases it is not clear-cut. Both cancer and stroke become more common in older individuals, and therefore there is a natural overlap between the two conditions.

Some studies published in the neurological literature suggest that stroke can occur in a variety of cancers; 47% of patients presenting with stroke and an underlying malignancy had cancer that had already spread (metastasized). Half of the strokes were related to emboli (mobile clots), and the other half were thrombotic or clots forming within the vessel. Some studies have estimated that approximately 8% of patients dying with cancer had a stroke, although it is not known how many of these strokes are directly related to the cancer because patients can have strokes with or without cancer.

Table 3   Cancers associated with strokes

Lung	30%
Brain	9%
Prostate	9%
Breast	4%
Lymphoma	6%
Leukemia	6%
Gynecologic	6%
Bladder	6%
Gastro esophageal	6%
Other	20%

In some studies approximately 12% to 24% of strokes in patients with cancer are related to the cancer causing a clotting abnormality. Another significant number of strokes are caused by abnormalities on the heart valves known as marantic endocarditis. Marantic endocarditis refers to deposits of gelatinous sticky material with inflammation that can be seen with some cancers and can break off to cause strokes. Because most strokes in patients who have cancer are not directly related to the cancer, basic investigation for the cause of the stroke is warranted.

In some patients who have cancer the clotting system becomes deranged. This derangement causes both clotting and bleeding. Testing for these changes is important and includes D-dimer, which has been found to be elevated in 30% to 90% of patients with cancer, depending on the extent of the cancer. D-dimer alone is not specific for cancer, but its elevation raises suspicions that deserve further investigations. D-dimer is a byproduct of the breakdown of fibrin, which is an important element in the clotting cascade.

Treatment of the cancer is the most important element in reducing the potential blood-related complications. In patients with strokes related to cancer, the problem is often associated with a widespread derangement of the clotting system causing both bleeding and clotting. Therefore, in some cases, patients may suffer from both a hemorrhage (bleed) and an ischemic stroke. The treatment of these complications is difficult, but a careful approach to treatment with supplements to restore some of the clotting proteins as well as blood-thinning medications may have to be used simultaneously.

PART SEVEN

Hemorrhagic Stroke

What are the major causes of
intracerebral hemorrhages?

What factors contribute to worsening
of outcome in bleeds?

How do you treat bleeds?

More . . .

Several different types of hemorrhages (bleeds) occur within the brain and outside the brain. Outside the brain, epidural bleed occurs as a result of trauma and is not discussed further. Subdural bleed occurs under the covering of the brain but still outside the brain and can occur spontaneously or as a result of trauma; this condition also is not discussed in this book. In this section we concentrate on subarachnoid bleed, one that occurs on the surface of the brain and is usually the result of either trauma or a bleeding aneurysm, and intracerebral bleed, which is a bleed inside the brain. There are two different types of intracerebral bleeds: primary and secondary. A primary bleed is one that occurs from damaged arteries from hypertension or other processes. A secondary bleed may occur because an ischemic stroke (a stroke that occurs from local absence of blood flow from obstruction of an artery) "transforms," or turns into, a bleeding stroke; this **hemorrhagic transformation** is also discussed later in relation to worsening in ischemic stroke (see p 139).

Hemorrhagic transformation

Occurs when an ischemic stroke becomes hemorrhagic.

40. What are the major causes of intracerebral hemorrhages?

Intracerebral hemorrhage occurs as a result of weakening in the wall of the artery, which then leaks blood inside the brain. The weakening of the wall may occur from a variety of problems but is most commonly associated with hypertension, especially in patients between the ages of 40 and 70 years. Hypertensive changes can create changes in the artery with small blebs in the wall of the artery known as Charcot-Bouchard aneurysm. In patients over age 60, amyloid angiopathy is an important contributor to bleeding. This condition is the result of deposition of amyloid protein in the wall of the artery, resulting in weakening of the wall and subsequent bleeding. Hypertensive changes in the artery and amyloid deposition results in brittle arteries and prevents the natural physiological mechanisms of the artery from responding to limit the bleeding. The use of blood-thinning medications such as warfarin is also associated with a higher risk of bleeding. In younger patients the cause of bleeding is likely to be related to venous–arterial malformations or **cavernous angioma**. Bleeding disorders can occur because of clotting abnormalities in patients with severe infections or advanced cancer. Certain drugs have also been associated with intracerebral hemorrhage.

Bleeds caused by hypertension have predilection to occur in specific locations in the brain. The size and the location of the bleed determine the symptoms and ultimate recovery. One of the common places for intracerebral bleed to occur is the pons, which is part of the brainstem. This area of the brainstem is a major structure that acts as a control center for eye movements and is a major highway carrying motor, sensory, and balance information. Another common area for bleeds is the putamen, an important part of the motor system that is geographically close to the motor fibers; therefore a hemorrhage in that area can cause paralysis on the opposite side of the body. The third common location for an intracerebral hemorrhage is the thalamus, which is a major relay center for sensory information and memory.

The location of the bleeds is a reflection of vulnerable arteries that become damaged when receiving unusually high pulsating influx of blood. Structures in the brain that can diffuse large pulse pressure by other intermediary arteries, as may occur in the superficial parts of the brain, are less vulnerable to damage induced by elevated blood pressure. However, the superficial areas are affected by other processes such as amyloid angiopathy that can cause bleeds.

The diagnosis of a bleed is usually accomplished with a CT. Acute blood looks bright on a CT. Although MRI can also detect blood, MRI is not as readily available in some places. MRI is a better test to look at older bleeds as well. A combination of CT and MRI may be necessary to help find the etiology of the bleed. Because of the presence of blood, underlying problems, such as vascular malformation or a tumor,

Cavernous angioma

Vascular malformation that can bleed or cause transient ischemic attack-like symptoms.

Bleeds caused by hypertension have predilection to occur in specific locations in the brain. The size and the location of the bleed determine the symptoms and ultimate recovery.

Hemorrhagic Stroke

may not be easy to see, and a repeat imaging with and without contrast may be necessary. Under some circumstances, where there is only an isolated bleed in someone without risk factors such as hypertension, one has to be concerned about underlying brain tumor or vascular malformation. If appropriate, imaging of other parts of the body may help define an underlying malignancy. In patients under age 45, it is important to consider underlying vascular malformations such as arterial–venous malformation or cavernous angioma. The former can be diagnosed sometimes on MRI and MRA. But traditional angiography is considered to be more helpful. A cavernous angioma can be difficult to diagnose in the acute state. Sometimes angiograms can demonstrate an associated large draining vein, which can be a hint. Repeating the imaging over a few months may be the only way to ultimately diagnose some of these lesions. To find out the reason for the hemorrhage it is important to look for any clotting abnormalities that may have been predisposed to the bleeding, and when appropriate a toxicology screen may be done to look for illicit drugs that may predispose to hemorrhages.

Although it was believed that hemorrhagic stroke has a better long-term outcome, the data are still sketchy. Rebleeding, especially in large bleeds, is one of the major reasons for worsening in hemorrhages; smaller bleeds were believed to have a better outcome than similarly sized ischemic strokes. The reason for the differences is that blood that does not destroy tissue simply seeps through the tissue, pushing structures around but not necessarily killing the tissue. After the acute period, the rate of medical complications and death is similar in both types of stroke.

41. What factors contribute to worsening of outcome in bleeds?

Patients with bleeds generally worsen in the first few days for a variety of reasons, including rebleeding, swelling, and medical complications. Swelling is common in any type of insult to the brain and is discussed in detail in relation to complications of stroke in a different section of this book (see p 135). Similarly, the medical complications are discussed in relation to ischemic stroke (see p 132) and therefore are not discussed here. Rebleeding is a feared early complication and occurs in 30% to 60% of patients, generally in the first 48 hours but rarely up to a week. Rebleeding occurs in 38% of patients in the first 3 hours after the onset of symptoms. Patients with large bleeds are more likely to rebleed. Overall, the mortality rates of cerebral hemorrhage in the first 30 days ranges from 40% to 60%.

The vessels in my brain were severely compromised due to the unknown assault on my brain. Given my precarious condition, I was monitored in ICU for a week, while they tried to unravel what had caused the bleed. I could not have any foods that contained caffeine or medicines that could elevate my blood pressure. I was told that any strain—blowing my nose, straining on the toilet, or laughing might cause another bleed. I was in emotional limbo: I needed to cry, albeit privately, but I also wanted to joke and laugh as a coping mechanism. The fear of inducing another bleed also left me constipated for over nine days.

42. How do you treat bleeds?

Intracerebral hemorrhage continues to be one of the most difficult conditions to manage in neurology. The high rates of medical complications and death associated with this condition and the lack of definitive treatment are very frustrating to physicians, patients, and families. The leading cause of worsening outcome in bleeds is the acute rebleeding; 38% of patients show worsening of the bleed within 3 hours. The increase in the size of the bleed, however, may continue in more than 70% of patients over the next 24 hours. Similar to ischemic strokes, hemorrhagic strokes develop swelling, which can be temporarily managed with osmotic diuretic agents such as mannitol. Mannitol can help to decrease the swelling by eliminating extra fluid from normal parts of the brain. Hy-

Rebleeding occurs in 30% of patients in the first 3 hours after the onset of symptoms.

Hemorrhagic Stroke

perventilation can also help decrease the swelling but, again, only temporarily; this topic is discussed further under ischemic stroke. Removing the bleed surgically is controversial, and multiple surgical approaches and techniques have been attempted depending on the location of the bleed. Deep bleeds such as in the basal ganglia and the pons cannot be reached without damaging normal brain structures in the way, whereas superficial bleeds in the cortex are easier to reach. Some studies have demonstrated that by removing the bleed with microscopic instruments and with infusion of the clot-busting drug tissue plasminogen activator it is possible to reduce the size of the bleed, but it is not clear if this approach leads to improved neurological outcome. In the appropriate setting, the placement of a ventricular drain may help decompress the brain and clear blood from the ventricles.

Overall, studies have demonstrated slightly better outcome with surgery, 26.1% versus 23.8%, but survival rates appear to be similar in surgically and medically treated patients (International Surgical Trial in Intracerebral Hemorrhage, 2005). Subgroup analysis suggests that large hemorrhages, severe neurological deficits at presentation, and older age predict universally poor outcome. Other factors that contribute to poor outcome include blood in the ventricle and enlargement of the ventricle, suggesting obstruction of flow of the spinal fluid from blood. Overall, 20% of patients later recover to become independent. However, some evidence suggests that superficial bleeds do better with surgery than with medical treatment, 49% versus 37%. Neurosurgeons generally agree that significant bleeds in the cerebellum need to be removed to improve outcome. The cerebellum is located in the back and bottom part of the brain near the brainstem and near spinal fluid drainage system, therefore expanding bleeds can potentially compress adjacent structures leading to death. But there is no general agreement on evacuation of other bleeds. This problem sometimes creates conflicts between neurologists and neurosurgeons as to the appropriateness of surgical intervention in some cases.

Medical treatment using activated factor VII may become an important element in the treatment of intracerebral bleeds. Activated factor VII is an initiator of clotting. Once activated, factor VII binds to the surface of platelets and generates aX, which in turn induces surface thrombin formation and triggers the clotting cascade. Because activated factor VII works in the presence of tissue factor, which is released by injured brain, it seems to have its primary effects at the site of the bleed. Manufactured forms of factor VIIa, known as recombinant factor VIIa (rFVIIa), have been used effectively in patients who have hemophilia. More recently, a safety study of rFVIIa used to treat intracerebral hemorrhage demonstrated a benefit in reducing the size of the hemorrhage when given within 4 hours of onset of hemorrhage. At 24 hours and based on repeat CT, patients who received placebo had an increase in the size of the bleed by 29%, whereas in patients receiving the rFVIIa the size of the bleed increased by 11% to 16% depending on the dose of drug. Mortality at 3 months was decreased by 29% in patients who did not receive rFVIIa and by 18% in those who received it. Because this drug induces clotting, it was not surprising to see increased risk of clotting, 7% in patients receiving the drug and 2% in patients receiving the placebo. The events were evenly distributed between venous clots, ischemic strokes, myocardial infarction, and pulmonary embolus. These data are very encouraging because this drug may prove to be effective in minimizing the damage from the bleed and improving outcome. Further studies are underway to understand the true risks and benefits of this drug.

43. How do you manage blood pressure in patients with a bleed?

It is not entirely clear that tight control of blood pressure can change the outcome from intracerebral hemorrhage. In patients who are admitted to the hospital with intracerebral hemorrhage, the blood pressure may be elevated for a variety of reasons. Because hypertension is the leading cause of bleeding in older patients, it is not surprising that some

Hemorrhagic Stroke

patients admitted with a bleed have an elevated blood pressure. The natural responses to large bleeds and the anxiety of being gravely ill can all result in an excessive elevation of blood pressure. Whether that elevation alone is contributing to worsening of the bleed or ultimately worsening of the outcome is unknown. Furthermore, it is not known how blood vessels react to bleeding and to elevation in blood pressure in individuals who already have problems with blood pressure. This uncertainty provides an opportunity for clinical studies. In the meantime, recommendations have been made to maintain systolic blood pressure below 180 mm Hg. After the acute phase of the bleed, it is important to closely monitor and treat "hypertension," because lowering the blood pressure by 10 mm Hg reduces the risk of another hemorrhage by half.

Excessive lowering of blood pressure can also be harmful to the brain with a stroke of any kind. After a stroke there are areas of the brain that are marginally alive, otherwise known as the penumbra. That area of brain potentially can be salvaged if we can optimize perfusion (the flow of blood) and limit the spillover of toxins from surrounding dead or dying brain tissue. Usually, a normal brain has the capacity to accommodate a wide range of blood pressure fluctuations due to "autoregulation." This autoregulation maintains perfusion of the brain tissue in spite of significant drops in blood pressure. There is also enough capacity in the blood vessel to absorb higher pressure. Autoregulation can only work within certain parameters, excessive elevation or drop in blood pressure can damage the arteries and the brain tissue. In patients with stroke, the arteries are damaged and so is the brain's ability to adjust to fluctuations in blood pressure. Unfortunately, research in this area has not helped in determining the optimal blood pressure control in cases of acute cerebral hemorrhage or in ischemic stroke. Some assumptions are made from indirect evidence that systolic blood pressure above 180 mm Hg can increase the risk of bleeding or rebleeding. Low blood pressure may lower the perfusion of marginal brain tissue to a critical point that results in cellular death. Small studies suggest a benefit to artificially increasing the blood pressure in ischemic stroke. A systolic blood pressure of 150 mm Hg may be a significant threshold below which neurological deterioration may occur. Therefore, the recommendations for both hemorrhagic and ischemic strokes are to maintain the systolic blood pressure around 150 mm Hg.

44. How common is bleeding from warfarin?

Warfarin (Coumadin) is a blood-thinning medication frequently used to help treat clots in veins and to help prevent strokes from atrial fibrillation. The major complication from the use of warfarin is bleeding. The risk of intracerebral hemorrhage while on warfarin increases by as much as five times. One study demonstrated that 18% of all cases of intracerebral hemorrhages admitted to the hospital occurred while patients were on warfarin. Although there is a trend for higher rate of bleeding with higher INR, most bleeds still occur when the INR is in the recommended range of 2.0 to 3.5. Expansion of the bleed is more likely to occur when the INR is excessively elevated. The location of bleed in those on warfarin versus spontaneous bleeds is similar, implying that bleeds under those circumstances affect arteries that are vulnerable to bleeding in the first place.

Because of the potential of expansion of the bleed, it is important to reverse the anticoagulant (inability to clot) effects of warfarin as soon as possible. This process can be difficult with no guidelines available. Obviously, discontinuation of warfarin is the first step, but the anticoagulant effects are usually not fully reversed for several days. Because the expansion of the bleed occurs in the first 24 hours, simply discontinuing warfarin alone does not reverse the effects quickly enough. Because warfarin acts by inhibiting vitamin K activities, giving additional vitamin K intravenously should help reverse the effects of warfarin; unfortunately, even the administration of vitamin K may not be sufficient to rapidly reverse the anticoagulation, because the benefit may not be realized for up to 24 hours. Fresh frozen plasma, a blood product that contains clotting factors, may also not become effective for more than 24 hours. More specific procoagulant drugs, such as prothrombin complex concentrate and factor VIIa concentrate, are faster acting, usually within 15 minutes. However, the disadvantages of these drugs are the potential for causing clots, a short half-life (effect does not last long), and cost.

In the acute period and after the intracerebral hemorrhage and the discontinuation of warfarin, there is a risk of recurring stroke. Some studies suggest that the risk of a recurring stroke in the initial 14 days is relatively small. The harder decisions are when to restart any form of anticoagulation, including subcutaneous heparin or warfarin after the patient suffers from a bleed. There are no studies to help determine the risks versus benefits of early re-anticoagulation.

When patients develop hemorrhagic complications from warfarin, it becomes difficult to justify restarting warfarin. But there are circumstances when this can be done safely. Clinical studies testing the effects of warfarin did not enroll patients with a history of bleeding problems. Small studies seem to suggest that the risk is not significantly elevated. But these studies do not provide enough data to be certain of the potential for complication. Some studies have suggested that the existence of significant "small vessel disease" (i.e., strokes in the deep part of the brain) or evidence of prior bleeds contributes to higher risk of rebleeding. It has been suggested that the risk of rebleeding after an initial intracerebral hemorrhage outweighs the benefits of anticoagulation with warfarin in patients who have atrial fibrillation. However, in patients with artificial valves, warfarin may be justifiable because of an otherwise exceedingly high risk of stroke without warfarin. The risk of rebleeding with the reintroduction of warfarin in patients with gastrointestinal bleed is unknown. However, if an underlying cause of bleeding can be identified and treated and no other sources of high-risk bleeding can be found, then restarting anticoagulation is reasonable.

45. What is an arterial–venous malformation?

These are abnormalities in arteries and veins that are inter-mingled to form a highly vascular collection of blood vessels with aneurysmal expansion and fragile connections. It is unknown how common **arterial-venous malformations (AVMs)** are in the general population, but estimates range from 1 to 2 per 100,000 individuals for all vascular malformations. Approximately 10% of patients become symptomatic from vascular malformations. The symptoms are the results of bleeding, enlargement, or "stealing" of blood from nearby structures; as a result presentations vary from severe headaches to transient ischemia and stroke-like symptoms to seizures. The most common presentation is a hemorrhage, followed by seizures. The risk of hemorrhage is estimated at 3% per year with significant medical complications and death. The risk of a recurrent hemorrhage in the first year after the initial hemorrhage is between 6% and 30%. However, because this is a fairly uncommon problem the true risk is still unknown, although clearly it is much higher than if the malformation never hemorrhaged. The presence of aneurysmal expansion and less developed venous drainage as well as certain locations such as near the ventricular system are important factors that may lead to higher risk of bleeding. If the arterial-venous malformation is asymptomatic, it is difficult to justify aggressive treatment because treatments are associated with potential neurological complications. Once symptoms occur, there are several options for intervention. If the hemorrhage is significant, it is important to try decompressing the brain by removing the blood and the malformation. If the bleeding is small, then the treatment may include a combination of interventional treatment to occlude major arterial feeders into

Arterial venous malformation (AVM)

Abnormal collection of arteries and veins that can bleed.

Hemorrhagic Stroke

the malformation, followed by surgical removal. Small arterial venous malformations may be treated with focused radiation. The latter approach may take years to reduce or obliterate the malformation. The location of the arterial venous malformation also dictates the type and level of interventions. Deep locations (i.e., those that are difficult to reach surgically such as the basal ganglia or the brainstem) or malformation near the motor cortex or in language areas may best be treated with nonsurgical techniques. Placing glue and coils in the arterial venous malformation is a promising nonsurgical technique but on its own has only been shown to be curative in a small number of cases. Even with this less-invasive technique, hemorrhaging and other neurological complications can occur. A combined approach is often necessary, which includes the use of presurgical gluing followed by resection.

Placing glue and coils in the arterial venous malformation is a promising nonsurgical technique.

Because of the altered blood flow dynamics within the malformation, which often has existed for many years, severe brain swelling and hemorrhaging may occur during treatment. Some physicians have recommended that, when possible, the arterial venous malformation should be treated in stages to allow the brain and vessels to adjust to the new blood flow. However, other physicians believe that the bleeding is simply due to obstruction of blood flow through the arterial system to some extent, but more importantly the venous system. When blood flow is obstructed in the venous system, normal outflow from either residual arterial feeders or normal arterial feeders into the venous bed is hindered, causing buildup of pressure in relatively fragile blood vessels. This can cause leakage of blood or a frank hemorrhage in addition to swelling in the brain. Although the best approach to treatment is still debated, it is important to approach treatment options cautiously and to consider the staged approach but also to make sure that the treatment is done by physicians with the reputation and experience in this field.

Initially, a burst AVM was thought to be the cause. I remember feeling relieved that there was potentially a definitive diagnosis, but had concerns for my son and siblings, as this is a hereditary condition. To confirm the diagnosis, I needed an angiogram (the first of three I would have in six months). I learned that having a burst AVM would not be a good thing, as it is often fatal, but good or bad, I wanted an explicit diagnosis. After the angiogram and an MRI, the AVM was ruled out, and cerebral vasculitis became the prime suspect.

46. What is a cerebral cavernous angioma?

This is a different form of vascular malformation made out of a cavity (cavernous) with abnormal vessels (angioma). Cerebral cavernous malformation or angioma (CCM) has been shown to have two forms, an inherited form and a sporadic form (noninherited). Patients may have either a single lesion, usually in the sporadic form, or multiple lesions in the familial form. The inherited condition is not always predictable. There are three genes that have been identified in the familial forms, *CCM1/KR1T1, CCM2/MGC4607,* and *CCM3/PDCD10.* Familial CCM has been shown in large clusters in Hispanic-American families. Screening for these genetic abnormalities is available in special laboratories. Imaging studies of the brain may suffice, however, in screening families. The heterogeneous genetic expression has been studied to some extent, and it appears that the different genes may have some predictive value in assessing the risk of hemorrhage. For example, CCM1-affected individuals have fewer bleeds than other individuals with different forms of the mutation. These differing clinical expressions may be of little use because on an individual basis the risk of bleeding is still present.

Clinically, patients with this condition may present with headaches, transient ischemic-like spells, seizures, and other neurological symptoms. Many cavernous angiomas bleed slowly. Initial bleeds may cause no symptoms, because the bleed may be contained in the "cave." When the blood expands outside the cavity it begins to cause symptoms, such as seizures or transient ischemic attack-like episodes. If the bleeding is large, then the presentation is similar to that discussed in the intracerebral hemorrhage section (see p 62). It may be difficult to diagnose a cavernous angioma, because when the patient presents with an intracerebral hemorrhage the lesion may not be seen within the collection of blood. Additional MRIs/CTs need to be performed over time before a definite diagnosis can be made. Some of these cavernous lesions contain a large vein, which sometimes can be seen on imaging or angiograms. Cavernous malformations can also occur in the eye and spinal cord.

PART EIGHT

Subarachnoid Hemorrhage

What are the symptoms of
subarachnoid hemorrhage?

What is a warning leak?

How do you diagnose subarachnoid hemorrhage?

More . . .

Subarachnoid hemorrhage refers to the location of blood in areas around the brain, the subarachnoid space. The cause of bleeding is usually from either trauma or bleeding from an aneurysm. For the purposes of this book, we discuss aneurysms and not trauma. Aneurysms occur in specific areas of arteries, usually at branching points. It is estimated that approximately 5% or approximately 15 million people in the United States have asymptomatic aneurysms, whereas the number of patients who suffer from subarachnoid hemorrhage is 30,000 per year. These numbers suggest that aneurysms in most people do not rupture. However, once the aneurysm ruptures, there are many serious complications that can lead to strokes and death.

47. What are the symptoms of subarachnoid hemorrhage?

The initial symptoms of subarachnoid hemorrhage are usually a headache that may be associated with nausea, vomiting, disorientation, and other neurological deficits. The headache quality is fairly severe and reaches a maximal point rapidly. This headache is often described as "the worst headache ever." This usually prompts an evaluation in the emergency room. However, most headaches seen in the emergency room are not caused by subarachnoid hemorrhage or other serious neurological conditions, and many benign headaches can mimic the characteristics of subarachnoid hemorrhage. Ultimately, and once a subarachnoid hemorrhage occurs, it may result in additional neurological problems, including swelling of the brain and vasospasms. The **spasms** can lead to ischemic strokes.

Spasms

Constriction of the blood vessels, usually in reaction to inflammation or damage to the artery or chemical changes in the surrounding area, as may occur with subarachnoid hemorrhage.

An aneurysm can leak instead of burst.

48. What is a warning leak?

An aneurysm can leak instead of burst. The leakage is often referred to as a "sentinel" bleed or warning leak. In one retrospective study published in 1994, of 148 patients presenting with symptoms suggesting a sentinel subarachnoid hemorrhage, 25% were ultimately diagnosed as having a subarachnoid hemorrhage. Another study in 2005 reviewed the history and outcome in 214 patients who where diagnosed and treated for subarachnoid hemorrhage; 31% had symptoms suggesting a warning leak that preceded the subarachnoid hemorrhage by a median of 11 days. In this review it was suggested that patients with warning leak presented in a worse neurological status and had earlier spasms, but the outcome at 22 months was no different between the group with the warning leak and those without.

Although the characteristics of a warning leak may help guide further workup, in patients with a history of headaches sometimes differentiating between new types of a headache that reflects significant neurological disease and a variant of the baseline headache can be difficult. Furthermore, because approximately 30,000 patients suffer from a subarachnoid hemorrhage a year and there are over 27 million people with benign headaches, many patients with benign headaches can suffer from a subarachnoid hemorrhage and some patients with subarachnoid hemorrhage suffer from benign headaches. Furthermore, the limitations of the noninvasive testing (i.e., the inability to detect certain sized aneurysms on CTA and MRA) and the overlap between two disease processes inevitably lead to missed diagnosis.

49. How do you diagnose subarachnoid hemorrhage?

As discussed earlier, subarachnoid hemorrhage implies that bleeding has occurred in the subarachnoid space. In this case the blood is usually detected on a CT, which has over 95% sensitivity. If the CT does not demonstrate blood, then a spinal fluid analysis, usually by lumbar puncture, is the next step in the diagnosis if a subarachnoid hemorrhage is clinically suspected. An MRI can also see blood, but sensitivity and specificity of MRI in the detection of acute blood in the subarachnoid space has not been rigorously evaluated. MRI does not replace spinal fluid tests, however, because there appears to be a need for a minimum amount of residual blood necessary before MRI can detect the subarachnoid hemorrhage. In one study the rate of positive MRI tests when CT was negative but lumbar puncture was positive was only 16.7%.

Once a subarachnoid hemorrhage has been detected, finding the source of the bleed is important. Two noninvasive tests, MRA and CTA, can be helpful. Both tests have advantages and disadvantages. A study of MRA compared with cerebral angiography in patients with a recently ruptured aneurysm suggested that a contrast-enhanced MRA is very accurate in localizing the aneurysm and in characterizing it. But in pre-symptomatic aneurysms (i.e., no bleed) MRA is still inferior to cerebral angiography. Aneurysms smaller than 3 mm can be missed on MRA. CTA provides another tool to help diagnose aneurysms. Some studies on the utility of CTA in detecting aneurysm suggested that the sensitivity is 90%, whereas other studies suggested that the sensitivity is higher around 97%, but small aneurysms less than 4 mm are more likely to be missed on CTA.

50. What is the risk of bleeding from an aneurysm?

Depending on the history, risk factors, location and size of the aneurysm, there are different degrees of risks associated with bleeding. Table 4 is a simplified summary of the results of a study published in 1998 that assessed factors associated with rupturing of aneurysm (The International Study of Un-ruptured Intracranial Aneurysms Investigators). This study divided individuals into two groups.

Group 1 included patients with no history of ruptured aneurysm but found to have an aneurysm by imaging study done for evaluation of other neurological conditions. Group 2 included patients who had already suffered from a rupture of an aneurysm but had another asymptomatic aneurysm.

This study revealed differences in the two groups, as detailed in Table 4. In addition to size, in group 1 (no bleed) larger aneurysms in the tip of the basilar artery, posterior cerebral artery, or posterior communicating artery were more likely to rupture. However, in group 2 (with bleed) the only important high-risk variable was location in the tip of the basilar artery. The death rate with ruptured aneurysm was on the average of 66%—83% in group 1 and 55% in group 2. The differences in the two groups in death rate are likely to be related to selection bias. Surgical outcome seems to indicate a high morbidity and mortality in both groups. The conclusion from this study was that it was unlikely that surgery improves outcome in individuals with aneurysms smaller than 10 mm and no history of subarachnoid hemorrhage. It appears that patients with prior history of aneurysmal rupture are at a higher risk of having a subarachnoid hemorrhage from another asymptomatic aneurysm.

Table 4   Factors associated with aneurysm rupture

Group 1			
Aneurysm size	% rupture per year	Mortality when ruptured	Morbidity and mortality with treatment
Less than 10 mm	0.05%	83% (for large and small)	15.7% (for large & small)
More than 10 mm	1.0%		
Group 2			
Aneurysm size	% rupture per year	Mortality when ruptured	Morbidity and Mortality with treatment
Less than 10 mm	0.5%	55% (for large and small)	13.6% (for large & small)
More than 10 mm	1.0%		

Subarachnoid Hemorrhage

Another study published in 2003 demonstrated a clear preference of bleeding from aneurysms located in arteries of the posterior circulation and in patients with aneurysms greater than 7 mm, or one-fourth of an inch. The percent of bleeding over 5 years is summarized in Table 5.

Table 5   Percentage of bleeding from aneurysms (over 5 years)

	Size in mm (26 mm = 1 inch)			
	7 mm	**7–12 mm**	**13–24 mm**	**> 25 mm**
Anterior circulation	0%	2.6%	14.5%	40%
Posterior circulation	2.5%	14.5%	18.4%	50%

The anterior circulation includes the internal carotid artery (ICA), anterior communicating artery (Acom), anterior cerebral artery (ACA), and middle cerebral artery (MCA). The posterior circulation includes the basilar artery (BA), posterior communicating artery (Pcom), and posterior cerebral artery (PCA).

51. What are the risk factors that cause an aneurysm to bleed?

Some studies have tried to address this question. The two major factors that appear to be consistent are that larger aneurysms and those located in the posterior circulation greatly increased the risk of bleeding. Other studies using serial imaging studies of nonbleeding aneurysms or examination of aneurysm at autopsy demonstrated that the rate of growth of the aneurysm was associated with increased risk of bleeding. The average size of growing aneurysms that ruptured was approximately 11 mm. The rate of growth of aneurysms varied in this population that was followed for approximately 18 years. In some patients the aneurysm grew by 1 mm, whereas in others the aneurysm grew by more than 3 mm. The risk of developing a subarachnoid hemorrhage in this population of patients was 1.3% per year. Smoking was a significant risk factor linked to the risk of growth of the aneurysm. Also revealed was that many patients in this study, 17%, developed new aneurysms that were not present on initial angiographic studies. Patients who were at the highest risk of developing new aneurysms were more likely to be females who were currently smoking. The rate of developing a subarachnoid hemorrhage from a new aneurysm based on numbers from this study suggests that the risk is 11 per 100,000 per year. Therefore, at this time, factors that appear to guide follow-up protocols and treatment include the size, location, and rate of growth of the aneurysm. Other factors that contribute include smoking, female gender, and age greater than 60. Of interest, smoking has been shown to be a significant risk factor in many but not all studies. New experiments suggest that smoking can result in an imbalance in two chemicals, elastase and antitrypsin, which can cause weakening of the arterial wall and as a result contribute to rupture.

52. Do aneurysms smaller than 7 mm bleed?

It is clear that "small" aneurysms can bleed, but the risk of bleeding is exceedingly low compared with "large" aneurysms. The data summarized from recent studies suggest that the risk of bleeding from aneurysms smaller than 7 mm is 0.5% per year for the highest risk aneurysms in the posterior circulation (Table 5) and much smaller for patients of similar size aneurysm in the anterior circulation. Some studies have suggested that small aneurysms that bleed are often associated with hypertension and location in the posterior circulation. There is also some evidence to suggest that de novo aneurysms (aneurysms that form where none existed before) are more likely to bleed, possibly regardless of size. Ultimately deciding on when to intervene for an asymptomatic aneurysm must take into consideration several factors, including location of aneurysm, size of aneurysm, rate of growth, age, and risk factors for surgery.

53. Are aneurysms inherited?

There are inherited conditions, such as polycystic kidney disease, that can increase the risk of having intracranial aneurysms. However, equally important is the higher risk of having an aneurysm in individuals with two or more first-degree relatives (i.e., immediate family: sibling or parent) with an aneurysm. Screening studies of patients with first-degree relatives with aneurysms as well as in those with polycystic kidney disease suggest that the prevalence in both groups is relatively similar, at approximately 9%. Other studies have demonstrated that the incidence is as high as 20% and that there were no differences in ethnicity. Also, it appears that if the first screening test is unrevealing, that repeating the screening at 5 years results in a positive test in 7% of individuals. Furthermore, 16% of patients who were originally diagnosed as having an aneurysm developed new aneurysms. This is significantly higher than the prevalence of aneurysms in the general population, which is estimated at 0.5%. The numbers cited by the studies may not be completely accurate due to potential technical limitations and the threshold of available noninvasive tests. There are also concerns that patients with aneurysms in other arteries, such as the aorta, may have aneurysms in other parts of the circulation, including the brain. Individuals with a family history of aortic aneurysms should be screened for other aneurysms, and their family members should also be screened. Screening of first-degree relatives, however, has its critics, with some physicians advocating against screening. Analysis of impact of screening on treatment and treatment outcome suggest that to prevent one subarachnoid hemorrhage, 149 patients need to be screened and 298 would need to be screened to prevent one fatal subarachnoid hemorrhage. Furthermore, studies have demonstrated a significant psychological impact on individuals and families who are considered high risk for cerebral aneurysms and who require regular screening. The impact was greatest in individuals with a positive screen. Therefore, although screening in family members is reasonable, one must consider the impact of such screening and also the uncertainty about follow-up screenings and treatments.

54. Can you have a subarachnoid hemorrhage without an aneurysm?

Subarachnoid hemorrhage can occur as a result of trauma. Aneurysms that cause a bleed can occlude (close) and become undetectable on testing. A review study in 2003 of 806 patients who had a subarachnoid hemorrhage demonstrated that 86 had a negative angiogram on initial evaluation, 36 of whom had a condition known as perimesencephalic subarachnoid hemorrhage. This type of subarachnoid hemorrhage has not been associated with the usual arterial aneurysms or complications seen with subarachnoid hemorrhage. The remaining patients had repeated angiographies and other tests, such as MRI, MRA, CT, and/or CTA and traditional angiographies. Only a second angiography was able to find evidence of aneurysm in three cases that were initially negative, and in one case a third angiography was required. This study as well as other studies like it demonstrates the difficulties in finding an aneurysm in some cases, albeit not a common occurrence.

55. How is an aneurysm treated?

If an aneurysm requires treatment, then the options may include surgery or **coiling**. Both procedures can potentially accomplish the same goal—that is, to block blood flow to the aneurysm. There is some controversy about which aneurysm should be treated with surgery versus coiling. However, many neurosurgeons are moving away from surgery to coiling, because coiling is less invasive. There are some drawbacks to both procedures. Surgery requires extensive manipulation of the brain, which increases the risk for complications. During the surgery the surgeon must be careful not to damage the brain or nearby veins or arteries. Once the aneurysm is found, the surgeon places a clip at the base of the aneurysm to isolate it from the main artery. The clip is permanent and stays in the brain. Coiling is done through a catheter inserted through an artery in the groin. The catheter then is advanced to the area of the aneurysm and special metal coils are placed inside the

Coiling

Placement of metal coils in aneurysms to prevent the aneurysm from bleeding.

Subarachnoid Hemorrhage

aneurysm. These coils promote clots to form inside the aneurysm, and as a result the aneurysm is occluded (closed). The advantage of coiling is that location of the aneurysm becomes less problematic, because most aneurysms can be treated with the coiling procedures. Some aneurysms may not be amenable to such treatment or may require additional procedures. One drawback to coiling is that the constant pulsation of arterial flow near or at the base of the aneurysm can result in compacting the coiling deeper into the aneurysm and expose the walls of the aneurysm to high pressure flow. Because of this potential problem, patients are monitored closely by x-rays, brain scans, or repeat angiograms. A study in Europe (International Subarachnoid Aneurysm Trial) that compared clipping of aneurysm surgically versus coiling in patients who suffered from a subarachnoid hemorrhage demonstrated better 1-year outcomes in patients who were treated with coils than those treated surgically: 23.5% of patients were dead or dependent at 1 year in the coiling group versus 30.9% in the surgical group. Complications such as seizures were higher in the surgical group. However, one of the major drawbacks of coiling was the higher rate of recurrence of the aneurysm or rebleeding from the aneurysm, 17.4% versus 3.8%.

These data provide a good systematic review of possible differences between two treatment modalities. The interpretation from these studies is that coiling, although possibly associated with better long-term outcome, clearly has limitations. Proponents of surgery cite multiple other studies that demonstrated similar complication rates between the two procedures. Furthermore, some argue that other complications associated with coiling are often underestimated, including silent strokes. The best way to make a decision about the treatment of the aneurysm is to receive treatment in a center with experience in both surgical repair and coiling. Under those circumstances the type of treatment is not dictated by what is available but rather by the best possible option for the patient.

56. How do you treat complications from subarachnoid hemorrhage?

There are several complications that occur in association with subarachnoid hemorrhage, including rebleeding, hydrocephalus, and vasospasms. Rebleeding is simply due to the instability of the aneurysm after an acute bleed, therefore resulting in a second bleed. Hydrocephalus is related to failure of the drainage of spinal fluid through normal channels due to the presence of blood that blocks normal circulation of fluid. Vasospasm is a dreaded complication that can cause strokes. Early clipping or coiling of the aneurysm prevents rebleeding, and hydrocephalus is treated with external drains. On the other hand, vasospasms are more challenging. Vasospasms lead to brain ischemia that if persistent can cause permanent damage to the brain. The spasms often occur 4 to 12 days after the hemorrhage and affect up to 70% of all patients who present with aneurysmal bleed. Infarcts are present in at least 36% of patients and frequently lead to worse outcome or death. However, spasms may not be the only reason for decreased blood flow and infarcts. Using xenon brain imaging to measure regional cerebral blood flow demonstrated, in a significant number of patients, global reduction in cerebral blood flow that did not correspond to focal areas of spasm. This important observation suggests that treatment modalities need to take into account other mechanisms, aside from spasms that contribute to cerebral ischemia. Future research in this area is critical if we are to change the outcome from this disease.

The cause of vasospasms remains a mystery. However, studies suggest that there are multiple factors generated by the blood in the subarachnoid space or by the lining of the arteries that act to cause spasms. The consequences of these changes often can be devastating to the brain. Pathologically, vessels are found to be blocked with clumps of platelets and white blood cells, which result in brain ischemia. However, even in patients who recover after subarachnoid hemorrhage and spasms, the vessels undergo long-term structural changes most likely compromising their natural abilities to adjust to changes in blood flow.

57. How do you monitor for spasms?

Transcranial Doppler (TCD)

An ultrasound used to evaluate flow inside the head.

Current methods for monitoring spasms include the use of **transcranial Doppler (TCD)** and angiography. The latter technique is the most sensitive but is invasive. TCD is a noninvasive technique but with an average sensitivity of 75%. As is the case with vascular ultrasound, TCD looks at flow velocities. It is like listening to the flow of water in a hose: The ear may pick up changes in the sound of water that reflect increased or decreased flow. The ultrasound performs the same task as the ear but translates sound into pictures with waveforms. Several issues can impact the accuracy and interpretation of TCD. Although parameters help determine normal velocities from those consistent with spasm, those parameters range widely for the anterior circulation, whereas parameters for the posterior circulation have not been studied as extensively. Technical limitations that prevent ultrasound measurement of certain vessels are common and the introduction of induced hypertension and hypervolemic (increase fluid circulation) treatment can cause significant false-positive reading for spasms. Furthermore, spasms in smaller arteries cannot be measured by TCD. Therefore there is a significant need to establish better monitoring techniques.

58. How do you treat spasms?

Preventative treatment of spasms using nimodipine is strongly recommended. Nimodipine acts to block calcium channels and therefore prevents the activation of substances that can result in narrowing of the arteries, or may simply increase blood flow from unaffected arteries.

Once spasms are detected, there is an aggressive attempt to increase blood flow to areas suffering from ischemia. Increasing blood flow is accomplished via "triple-H" therapy: hypertension, hypervolemia, and hemodilution. This can be done in a variety of ways including infusing large amount of fluids or special solutions and/or by the administration of medications that artificially elevate the blood pressure and increase cardiac output. This technique has been used for over 20 years, but surprisingly there has only been one prospective randomized study of 30 patients. There are potentially many complications related to this treatment, including fluid overload in the heart and lungs, heart attacks, hyponatremia (decrease in sodium levels), swelling in the brain, and infections related to catheter use. It is also clear from available studies that despite triple-H therapy, almost half of the patients continue to have spasms or experience strokes. Other treatments for spasms, such as the use of angioplasty to open a spastic vessel, are used under some circumstances.

PART NINE

Vasculitis

What is giant cell arteritis?

What is primary central nervous system vasculitis?

Can other inflammatory diseases cause
central nervous system vasculitis?

More . . .

Vasculitis is a generic term referring to inflammation of the blood vessels. Many different conditions are classified as vasculitis, including giant cell arteritis, Takayasu's arteritis, primary central nervous system angiitis, human immunodeficiency virus (HIV)-associated vasculitis or vasculopathy, sarcoid, lupus, and a variety of other inflammatory diseases discussed in this section. The exact triggers for this disease are unclear, but some autoimmune mechanism is clearly important in developing this disorder. An exaggerated immune reaction to infections has been postulated as an important element in initiating the inflammation. Infections of the brain and the meninges (covering of the brain) with such pathogens as meningococcus and pneumococcus can cause severe inflammation of the vessels, leading to strokes. For example, *Listeria* can cause inflammation of the vessels and the brain with predilection to the brainstem. Syphilis, although is a less common cause for vasculitis in the United States, continues to be a concern in many countries as well as in patients with HIV. Fungal infections with *Cryptococcus, Histoplasma, Aspergillus,* and *Mucor* need to be considered as triggers for vasculitis in the appropriate setting. Viruses such as West Nile virus and varicella (chickenpox) have also been reported to cause vasculitis. Treatment of this disease requires long-term immune suppression.

59. What is giant cell arteritis?

The most common vasculitis seen in neurology is "giant cell arteritis" or "temporal arteritis." This condition was first described by Bayard Horton in 1932 and is therefore sometimes also referred to as Horton's disease. The prevalence of this disease increases in individuals over the age of 50 and has been estimated to occur in 30 to 200 per 100,000 individuals. There is a tendency for the disease to occur in individuals from Northern Europe and the Northern parts of the United States. It is very uncommon to see this disease in individuals from Asian or African descent. Approximately 40% of patients with giant cell arteritis suffer from a more diffuse inflammatory condition known as polymyalgia rheumatica.

Giant cell arteritis often results in inflammation of a branch of the external carotid artery, the temporal artery, hence temporal arteritis. The initial symptoms are directly related to involvement of the temporal artery with accompanying headaches, malaise, fevers, scalp tenderness, and pain with chewing. As the condition progresses, it often involves other arteries, including the ophthalmic artery. Involvement of the ophthalmic artery can lead to occlusion of the artery and subsequent blindness. However, this condition can extend to other parts of the vascular tree, including the carotid, the vertebral arteries, the aorta, and even the coronary arteries. Strokes may occur in this condition during the acute stage of the disease or few months after initiation of treatment. Putative diagnosis of this condition is based on symptoms, findings on examination, and elevated erythrocyte sedimentation rate/C-reactive protein. The definite diagnosis is obtained by a biopsy of the temporal artery, which typically demonstrates large inflammatory cells in the wall of the artery. Treatment of this condition requires long-term use of steroids. Some retrospective studies suggests that the use of antiplatelet agents or blood-thinning medication may also help in preventing thrombotic complications from this disease. The cause of the inflammation is unclear. In one study DNA analysis in specimen with confirmed giant cell arteritis demonstrated the presence of herpes simplex virus, but other studies failed to demonstrate DNA of herpes, cytomegalovirus, and Epstein-Barr virus. Some reports have suggested a higher prevalence of malignancies in patients with giant cell arteritis. The malignancies include gastrointestinal, blood, and lymph node. The treatment is with initial high-dose steroids, followed by a maintenance dose up to 2 years. Some have advocated intravenous high-dose steroids for 3 days followed by administration of oral prednisone of 40 to 60 mg/day. Because long-term use of steroids is associated with significant side effects, it is best to taper the steroids as soon as possible. The timing for the tapering is unknown but relies on a combination of clinical relapse and rise in the erythrocyte

Vasculitis

sedimentation rate. During tapering, 60% of patients experience relapse. Some case reports have suggested efficacy of non–steroid-based drugs such as cyclosporine A, which has been shown to be beneficial in small studies. A combination treatment with prednisone and methotrexate may reduce relapses compared with prednisone alone but does not obviate the use of steroids.

Another interesting vasculitis that contrasts with giant cell arteritis is Takayasu's arteritis. This disease is seen in younger women and is generally found in individuals of Asian descent and in South America. The disease affects the larger arteries such as aorta and its branches such as the subclavian and the carotid arteries. This results in narrowing of the arteries, causing strokes. This condition has been associated with tuberculosis. Although steroids are used in the treatment of Takayasu's arteritis, it is not as beneficial for long-term treatment.

60. What is primary central nervous system vasculitis?

Primary central nervous system vasculitis is an exceedingly rare condition. The brain is the only organ involved in this disease. Patients may present with confusion, strokes, headaches, and seizures. Central nervous system vasculitis involves small- and medium-sized arteries in the brain. Another possibly related condition that involves smaller vessels is Susac syndrome, which affects the deep white matter of the brain, the retina (eye), and the cochlea (hearing part of the inner ear). This disorder primarily affects young females and can mimic multiple sclerosis. Most patients present with confusion and fluctuating levels of alertness as well as fluctuating hearing and vision.

The diagnosis of vasculitis is often difficult to make, with some cases more indolent than others. The inflamed arteries can sometimes be visualized on an angiogram as "beaded" or "hypersegmented" or "string of pearls" or "link of sausages."

However, the appearance on an angiogram is not specific or sensitive. In one study, 38 patients underwent angiography to help with the diagnosis of angiitis followed by brain and leptomeningeal (covering of the brain) biopsy. Fourteen of 38 had typical appearing angiogram for angiitis, but none had angiitis by biopsy. Other diagnoses were made in 6 of the 14 patients, but in the remaining 8 the findings were non-diagnostic. Biopsy was positive in 2 of 24 who had a normal angiogram. Usually, the spinal fluid is abnormal with increased white blood cell counts, elevated proteins, and normal glucose; however, that test alone is not specific. Therefore, for now, the most specific and sensitive test is a biopsy of the brain and the meninges.

The angiogram that I had following the brain surgery to evacuate the blood showed that the large and small vessels in my brain appeared constricted like 'sausage links' and that the vessels had a berry-like appearance. There was no apparent reason for the condition of my brain, leaving the radiology team, as well as the neurology team perplexed. A rheumatologist diagnosed me with cerebral vasculitis, a very rare condition. I was told that vasculitis usually presents in the lower larger organs. I had an ultrasound of my lower organs as well as a second angiogram later to explore the lower organs. No other organs appeared to be affected. I was told that cerebral vasculitis, while incurable, can be treated into remission through high doses of the steroid, Prednisone and the chemotherapy, Cytoxan. My understanding was that this combination would suppress my immune system to arrest what was attacking my body. Although all the tests pointed to cerebral vasculitis, the only way to confirm this diagnosis would be to do a brain biopsy. I was willing to move forward because I wanted that definitive diagnosis, but we had to do our due diligence. A brain biopsy is brain surgery, with all the attendant risks. As we probed deeper, we found out that the biopsy could return negative results, but I could possibly still have the disease. The sampling could be removed from a 'quiet' area of my brain, yet the disease could exist in another portion of the brain. The thought of turning my head into a colander so some doctor's diagnosis could be confirmed lost its appeal. I decided to forgo the biopsy because I was already puzzled and didn't want more inconclusive information.

61. Can other inflammatory diseases cause central nervous system vasculitis?

There are many other systemic conditions that can sometimes present with neurological difficulties, including polyarteritis nodosa, hypersensitivity vasculitis, Behçet's disease, Wegener's granulomatoses, Churg-Strauss syndrome, Kawasaki's disease, lupus, and sarcoidosis. These are rare disorders with incidence rates from 2 to 10 per 1 million individuals. Some of these disorders present with primary involvement of the central nervous system, whereas others involve the central nervous system at a later phase in the disease process.

Although it is difficult to discuss the details of each disease entity in this book, here are some interesting observations on some of the diseases. Behçet's disease affects the brain and the spinal cord and can cause clots in the venous system of the brain as well as the formation of aneurysms and increased pressure inside the head. Behçet's disease is associated with inflammation within the eyes, genital ulcers, and abnormal lesions in the lungs, intestines, and the heart. Polyarteritis nodosa and Wegener's granulomatoses can affect the nerves as well as the brain and the spinal cord. The presentations of these disorders may not be obvious and include isolated painful nerve involvement, encephalopathy (confusion/lethargy), or dysfunction of a cranial nerve, such as facial paralysis, in combination with abnormalities in eye movements. Specific infections have been associated with some of these disorders. For example, polyarteritis nodosa has been associated with hepatitis B and C infections. The diagnosis of these disorders can be difficult. A blood test for antineutrophil cytoplasmic antibodies is positive in Churg-Strauss syndrome, Wegner's granulomatoses, and microscopic polyangiitis. Additional clinical and imaging evidence can help narrow down the condition. The treatment for these diseases requires the use of immune suppression with drugs such as cyclophosphamide.

62. Can sarcoidosis cause strokes?

Sarcoidosis is a systemic inflammatory disease with neurological involvement in approximately 5% of cases. The clinical presentation includes focal neurological symptoms and deficits, in addition to confusion and lethargy. Some of the symptoms are related to involvement of the hypothalamus and the pituitary gland, which control hormones and sodium levels. Ischemic and hemorrhagic strokes and focal narrowing of arteries have been reported, but they are very rare. The diagnosis of this condition requires a series of tests looking for abnormal lymph nodes, abnormal gallium scan, elevated angiotensin-converting enzyme level, clinical suspicion, and biopsy. Treatment is often difficult but includes the usual immunosuppressive drugs, sometimes in combination with blood-thinning medications, and when appropriate even interventions to open the arteries. As is the case with autoimmune diseases, the activity of the disease fluctuates, and therefore close monitoring of the patient's condition is warranted.

63. Can lupus cause strokes?

Lupus is another autoimmune disease, which is more common than sarcoidosis. Because this is a systemic disease, the neurological complications may be related to other conditions such as excessively elevated blood pressure due to involvement of the kidneys. It is unclear if the disease truly and directly affects the arteries of the brain, but in many patients there is also an underlying hypercoagulability due to the presence of lupus anticoagulant and abnormal functioning platelets. Lupus anticoagulant may coexist with other abnormal proclotting proteins. The anti-prothrombin antibody test is emerging as a more sensitive test for patients who are negative for anticardiolipin and lupus anticoagulant. The presence of more than one of these proteins significantly increases

Vasculitis

the risk of stroke. The use of blood-thinning medications can help reduce the risk of stroke, but the treatment does not eliminate the risk and treatment has not been studied systematically. In some cases patients develop a rare blood disorder known as thrombotic thrombocytopenic purpura, which can also cause strokes. Furthermore, some patients with lupus develop abnormal growth on the heart valves known as Libman-Sacks endocarditis as well as other cardiac abnormalities that can potentially be a source for strokes. As is the case with autoimmune diseases, controlled suppression of immunity is the mainstay of treatment. The presence of cardiac abnormalities and hypercoagulability may necessitate additional treatments to include blood-thinning medications or surgery.

Anticardiolipin antibodies are considered part of the antiphospholipid syndrome and do not require the clinical diagnosis of lupus. Some patients develop full-blown lupus many years after presentation with strokes or miscarriages. This disease often affects young people, and the initial presentation may be a miscarriage. Some patients develop skin changes, referred to as livedo reticularis; this is most visible on the abdomen and limbs with a spiderweb-like discoloration of the skin. Anticardiolipin antibodies on their own are often found in patients without clinical sequelae. Data on the consequences of having elevated anticardiolipin antibodies are still not clear. Some studies in stroke populations suggest that high titers of anticardiolipin IgG antibodies is an independent risk factor for first-ever stroke, even in older patients. Other long-term follow-up studies after having a stroke demonstrate no direct relationship for future risk of recurrence of stroke. Antibody testing can be misinterpreted, and multiple tests exist for anticardiolipin antibodies and related proteins. The amount and type of antibodies in the correct clinical setting are more significant than isolated elevation of the antibodies. Furthermore, antibody levels as well as the presence or the absence of some of these antibodies depends on many factors, including simple viral infections. Therefore before final conclusions are made regarding the relevance of these antibodies, repeating the test in 6 to 8 weeks should be done.

The recommendations for treatment of patients with anti-cardiolipin antibodies have continued to evolve and remain controversial. Some physicians advocate the use of aspirin in patients with no prior **thrombotic** events but persistently positive anticardiolipin antibodies. However, with thrombotic events or miscarriages more aggressive treatment may be needed to include blood-thinning medications with heparin/ warfarin and immunosuppressive drugs. The use of warfarin in combination with aspirin has also been advocated to treat high-risk patients with anticardiolipin antibodies who developed strokes. However, in 2004 a large study demonstrated no effect of aspirin versus warfarin on the risk of recurring stroke, heart attacks, deep vein thrombosis, or pulmonary embolus. Critics of this study suggest that a better benefit may have been observed if the level of anticoagulation with warfarin was higher. At this time, the need for anticoagulation with warfarin should be assessed on a case-by-case basis and in relation to other history of thrombotic events and coexisting risk factors.

Thrombotic

This refers to clotting of the blood within arteries or veins.

64. Can HIV cause strokes?

Human Immune Deficiency Virus (HIV) has been associated with a "vasculopathy," or damage to the vessels. This damage has been shown to lead to vascular changes that often are asymptomatic. The overall stroke and transient ischemia rates have been estimated at around 3%, higher than age-matched groups. There are many different causes for the ischemic events as may occur in the general population. However, HIV has been shown to be associated with a unique pathology in the vessel that predisposes the arteries to occlusive changes and aneurysm formation. The cause of the damage to the vessels is not entirely clear but includes deposition of immune

Vasculitis

response complexes; concurrent infections with pathogens such as cryptococcus, toxoplasmosis, tuberculosis, and varicella zoster; or even direct effects of the virus on the lining of the arteries.

PART TEN

Other Causes of Stroke

Can you have a stroke in the vein
instead of the artery?

What is arterial–venous dural fistula?

Can street drugs cause strokes?

More . . .

There are several other causes of stroke that do not fit in specific categories but are equally as important as the other types of strokes already discussed. In this section we discuss strokes caused by blockages in the vein instead of arteries, strokes associated with migraines and the use of oral contraceptives, strokes from sickle cell disease, and strokes due to inherited conditions such as CADASIL, to unusual vascular problems such as arterial venous fistulas, and strokes associated with street drugs. Many of these stroke syndromes can cause both ischemic and hemorrhagic strokes.

65. Can you have a stroke in the vein instead of the artery?

Formation of clots in veins is uncommon but can be devastating if a large vein, such as superior sagittal sinus, a big vein in the top of the brain, forms clots. When such a large vein is unable to provide drainage to the feeding vessels and even to the spinal fluid, pressure inside the brain rises and so does the pressure inside the feeding veins and arteries. As a result, one of the earliest signs of this problem is headaches, visual changes, and unsteadiness of gait, followed by seizures and strokes with hemorrhaging. This condition could be fatal if not recognized and treated promptly. Initial imaging studies such as a CT may not be diagnostic, and even MRI may not demonstrate obvious venous obstruction to help make the diagnosis. When clinically suspected, special imaging of the brain may be requested to include imaging of the veins, such as magnetic resonance venogram, which is not done routinely as part of a stroke evaluation.

Initial treatment includes controlling the seizures and lowering the intracranial pressure. Medications for the treatment of seizures can be given intravenously. Patients then need to be maintained on a specific amount of the medication on a daily basis to help prevent recurrence of these seizures. The high intracranial pressure can be managed with the use of osmotic diuretics such as mannitol, discussed in more detail in a different part of this book (see p 136). However, these are temporary measures, because the ultimate treatment is to reopen the vein to allow the reestablishment of normal arterial–venous circulation, which subsequently lowers the risk of strokes and decreases the swelling. Although blood-thinning medications such as heparin can be used to help prevent progression of the clot, this does not provide immediate recanalization of the vein. Therefore interventional procedures that can speed up the dissolving of the clot may be used if the patient's clinical situation warrants it. For example, in patients with clear worsening of symptoms, an intervention can be justified. The intervention includes placing a catheter in the large vein to mechanically disrupt the clot and to infuse clot-busting drugs, such as tissue plasminogen activator (t-PA). The amount of t-PA necessary to open the vein is unknown, and multiple infusions over several days may be necessary to improve flow. Because of occurrence of bleeding in venous strokes, there are concerns that the use of blood-thinning medications or clot-busting drugs may worsen the bleeding. In our experience with a handful of cases, this problem does not appear to be significant. Furthermore, considering the serious consequences of this disease, some risks are taken to help improve outcome. Not all cerebral vein thromboses are as serious. Some cerebral venous thromboses occur in smaller cortical veins. Usually, the symptoms include focal seizures, headaches, and neurological deficits. If the clots do not extend to the deeper and larger parts of the venous system and if the patient is clinically stable, then no aggressive intervention is necessary aside from the use of blood-thinning medications and medications to control seizures. Investigations for the underlying cause should be undertaken.

Venous clots usually have different causes from arterial clots. Many of the leading causes of venous clots are related to primary or secondary changes in the clotting system, including those occurring during pregnancy, and those associated with the use of estrogen and androgen supplements, dehydration, and the presence of a clotting disorder, especially mutation in factor V Leiden, although deficiencies in other clotting factors, such as protein C and S can also cause clotting in veins. It is believed that a combination of factors leads to the occurrence of venous clots. Studies have shown a higher prevalence of clotting disorders and use of estrogen (contained in oral contraceptives) in patients who develop cerebral venous thrombosis. In one study, 85% of patients with this problem were taking oral contraceptive versus 45% in age-matched controls subjects, and 19% had clotting disorder versus 7% expected in the general population. Another study demonstrated that a clotting disorder known as prothrombin gene mutation (factor II or *G20210A)*, was found in 20% of patients with cerebral thrombosis compared with 3% in control subjects. Furthermore, studies also demonstrated the effects of the "double-hit" concept, which refers to having a clotting abnormality, which by itself may not cause any problems, but when combined with another factor such as an oral contraceptive, the risk of cerebral vein thrombosis or other clotting disorder increases significantly. Other triggers for cerebral vein thrombosis include infections and malignancy, with either direct infiltration into the large veins or secondary to inducing a clotting abnormality.

Other triggers for cerebral vein thrombosis include infections and malignancy.

66. What is arterial–venous dural fistula?

Arterial–venous dural fistula, a very rare condition, is caused by an abnormal connection between an artery and a vein. An arterial–venous dural fistula can occur in the brain or in the spinal cord. In this condition, under high pressure, the veins receive blood from arteries, causing congestion in the venous system and increased pressure in the brain or the spinal cord. The pressure can be regional or global. In the brain the symptoms include headaches, difficulties with gait, blurred vision, spasticity, and Parkinson-like symptoms. In the spinal cord the symptoms seem to fluctuate and have a more classic presentation, with symptoms appearing with longer use and resolving with rest. Weakness in the lower extremities and bladder dysfunction are the major symptoms of spinal dural fistula. Arterial–venous dural fistula can be diagnosed on MRI and confirmed by angiography. It is best to treat this condition early when symptoms are minimal. Unfortunately, in the early stages of the disease it may be difficult to diagnose the condition clinically. Once the condition is identified, it is treated with either surgery or by embolization, or a combination of both. Treatment may be complicated by damage to the brain or the spinal cord that can impact recovery.

67. Can street drugs cause strokes?

Street drugs, such as methamphetamine, crack cocaine, and heroin, have been associated with strokes. In one study, 47% of patients under 35 years of age who had a stroke had no other identifiable cause but drug abuse. Strokes can result from an acute rise in blood pressure, causing bleeds inside the brain, vasculitis as a reaction to the drugs or contaminants within the drugs, and infectious material. Infarcts associated with drug use can result from heart infections (endocarditis) or from a reaction by the arteries, causing clots and occlusion of the arteries. The frequency of strokes related to street drugs is not known. Some studies have demonstrated that in young individuals with stroke there was a significant association of hemorrhagic stroke with the use of amphetamine, whereas cocaine abuse was associated with both hemorrhagic and ischemic strokes. The number one drug causing strokes in the young has changed over the years from cocaine to amphetamine.

68. Can sickle cell disease cause stroke?

Sickle cell disease is an inherited condition and common in individuals with African heritage or from regions of the Mediterranean. This is an inherited condition that results in the formation of red blood cells that contain abnormal hemoglobin, hemoglobin S. Having sickle cell disease implies that the individual inherited one sickle gene from each parent. However, there are many individuals who inherit

Street drugs, such as methamphetamine, crack cocaine, and heroin, have been associated with strokes. In one study, 47% of patients under 35 years of age who had a stroke had no other identifiable cause but drug abuse.

Other Causes of Stroke

only one sickle gene and therefore have the "trait" without ever developing complications. In sickle cell disease, the red blood cells' life span is reduced from 4 months to 2 weeks. The red blood cells also become stiff and misshaped, appearing like a sickle. The sickled blood cells block arteries, leading to organ damage. Sickle cell disease is a major cause of strokes in children and young adults. The risk for first stroke in patients with sickle cell disease is estimated at 10%. The rate of recurrence of stroke in some studies is as high as 90%. Strokes can be ischemic or hemorrhagic, related to large and/or small arteries. The cause of the strokes is multifactorial, including adherence of the diseased red blood cells to the lining of the arterial wall activating clotting cascade, damage to the wall of the artery, and development of aneurysmal dilatation.

Using transcranial ultrasound to measure the blood flow in the middle cerebral artery, a major artery supplying the brain, studies have demonstrated that in individuals with high velocities exceeding 200 cm/sec, there is a significantly higher risk for stroke. The STOP trial, Stroke Prevention Trial in Sickle Cell Anemia, demonstrated the benefits of regular transfusions with red blood cells in patients with high velocities by reducing the risk of first stroke from 10% per year to 1% per year. Studies on the discontinuation of transfusions have demonstrated that the stroke risk reverts back to pre-transfusion levels. One of the major side effects of frequent transfusions is iron overload, which can affect the function of the liver and other organs.

Another promising treatment is the use of hydroxyurea. This drug is approved by the U.S. Food and Drug Administration to help treat sickle cell disease. Hydroxyurea reduces the rate of sickling of the red blood cells, leading to fewer symptomatic attacks, and appears to reduce death rates, although its benefits in preventing strokes are unknown.

69. What is moyamoya disease?

This is an uncommon disease of the cerebral vessels that affects children and young adults. Moyamoya disease starts as an occlusive disease of the intracranial portions of the internal carotid arteries. Moyamoya has now been described in patients with different ethnic background, although the disease is still most commonly observed in Japan. Because of the chronic decrease in blood flow, the vessels secrete substances that allow for the proliferation of additional arteries to help perfuse regions of the brain in need of blood supply. The appearance of these arteries in the deep parts of the brain on angiography has been invariably described as a "puff of smoke," hence the Japanese name for the disease, moyamoya. The proliferation of arteries often results in vessels that are fragile and that can cause bleeding inside the brain. But because the vessels are also narrowed, transient ischemic attacks and strokes also occur. Generally, the middle cerebral artery is most commonly involved, but several studies have also shown that the posterior cerebral artery can be involved as well, especially in advanced stages of the disease. Most of the strokes occur in the territory of the middle cerebral artery and often occur in "watershed" areas between the middle cerebral artery and anterior cerebral artery. The cause of this disease is unknown, with an "idiopathic" (i.e., cause not found) form that often occurs in childhood and is primarily described in Japanese children and an atherosclerotic form that occurs in patients with risk factors for premature narrowing of certain vessels. However, in both forms of the disease the underlying pathophysiology that leads to such early and dramatic vascular changes remains speculative. Some investigators have proposed that the major cause of this disease is increased abnormal excitation of the wall of the arteries from adrenergic (contain adrenaline) nerve fibers originating from a nerve ganglion in the cervical spine. This excitation then leads to thickening of the blood vessel wall through other mechanisms that promote the production of collagen or collagen-like material within the wall of the artery, ultimately resulting in a decrease in blood supply.

Other Causes of Stroke

The treatment for this disease relies primarily on providing alternative blood supply to the deprived portion of the brain. This can be accomplished by a bypass, which entails taking an artery from the outside of the brain and connecting it to the inside of the brain. However, that is not always possible because a viable connection may not be found. An alternative is to place tissue or muscle rich in blood supply on the surface of the brain. These interventions do not provide immediate resolution to the problem, but over a period of 3 months they can help minimize the effects of compromised blood flow.

70. What is MELAS?

MELAS is an acronym for Mitochondrial Myopathy, Encephalopathy, Lactic Acidosis, and Stroke-like episodes. This is an inherited disorder of mitochondria (energy factory of the cell) and is due to mutation in mitochondrial DNA. Patients can develop transient ischemic attack-like symptoms, and many patients suffer from migraines. MRI demonstrates the predominance of stroke-like lesions in the posterior part of the brain. There is no known treatment for this disease.

71. Does radiation cause strokes?

Radiation effects may result in strokes, especially when radiation is applied to areas where arterial supply to the brain could be affected. Radiation can cause damage to the endothelium (lining of the artery) and premature development of atherosclerotic disease. The effects are often delayed, usually several years after the initial treatment. When the patient becomes symptomatic, treatment is generally similar to that applied to patients with primary atherosclerotic disease to the arteries. However many surgeons now prefer the use of stents on arteries affected by radiation instead of open surgery, due to the presence of adhesions around the arteries and due to the presence of other changes within the artery that makes surgery a less preferred option.

72. Do migraines cause strokes?

Migraine headaches are very common in the general population. In a subgroup of patients, stroke may become a significant complication of this disorder. Those migraine sufferers who appear to be at the highest risk of stroke are young women who suffer from migraine with aura, especially if they smoke and use oral contraceptives. Migraine with aura has been associated with a higher risk for strokes, ischemic and hemorrhagic, as well as cardiovascular events. The risk of stroke in women who suffer from migraines with aura is estimated at 3.8 additional cases per year per 10,000 women. Of interest, studies have also demonstrated an overall increase in all vascular events in patients with migraines with aura, with 18 additional major cardiovascular and cerebrovascular events per 10,000 women per year. What causes stroke in patients with migraines is not fully understood, but spasms in arteries causing narrowing and/or activation of platelets and promotion of inflammation could play a role in clot formation. It is unclear what treatments will limit the potential risk of stroke. The data suggest that smoking and the use of oral contraceptive should be eliminated in young women who suffer from migraines with aura. In addition, aggressive treatment of underlying risk factors such as hypertension, diabetes, and hypercholesterolemia should be undertaken. The use of a baby aspirin should also be recommended for those considered at high risk.

The risk of stroke in women who suffer from migraines with aura is estimated at 3.8 additional cases per year per 10,000 women.

73. Does taking oral contraceptives cause strokes?

The use of oral contraceptives has been linked to an increase in the rate of all types of vascular events, including strokes (Table 6). In the past, the risk of stroke was associated with the high amounts of estrogen contained in the first-generation oral contraceptive tablets. Epidemiological and animal studies over the past 10 years have, for the most part, demonstrated a higher risk for clotting events with use of oral contraceptives.

Table 6   Studies that have demonstrated a relationship between oral contraceptives and risk of strokes, ischemic and hemorrhagic

Study	Drug	Type of event	Risk of Treatment
Lancet. 1996; 348(9026):498–505	Estrogen/ Progestin	stroke	Higher risk with high estrogen Odds ratio 2.71 vs. 1.41
BMJ 1997; 315(7121):1502–4	high vs. low estrogen	stroke	Higher risk with high estrogen Odds ratio 4.4 vs. 3.9
Cephalgia 2000; 20(3):183–9	high vs. low estrogen	stroke	1/200,000 women years
JAMA 2003; 289(20): 1058–1062	Estrogen/ Progestin	stroke	8/10,000 more per year

Odds ratio is a term that refers to the "likelihood" of having an event. An odds ratio of 1 implies that the event is equally likely to occur in either groups, higher odds ratio in one group implies higher likelihood of having an event in that group.

These studies suggest that the overall risk of stroke is low in young women under the age of 35 who are currently not smoking and do not have other risk factors for stroke, including hypertension. In older individuals the risks need to be weighted against the benefits on an individual basis.

Several animal and human studies have suggested mechanisms in which estrogen can cause abnormal clotting. Increased platelet aggregation, increased levels of factor VII and D-dimer, and an increase in levels of inflammatory proteins as measured by C-reactive protein have all been shown to occur in patients taking estrogen. These effects have been seen in individuals taking estrogen for as little as 12 weeks. Even shorter term use of estrogen may be of concern. In spite of the fact that estrogen is broken down within a few days, some studies suggest a longer lasting effect because of an influence on certain functions of the clotting system. In one study using rats, a single dose of estradiol resulted in an increase in the level of estrogen, peaking at 7 days with levels returning to baseline at 4 weeks. In this study the investigators looked at clot formation in vessels in the lung, which peaked 21 days after the initial dose. The relevance of these findings to humans is unclear, although there have been reports of strokes in patients after taking a single high dose of estrogen formulation to prevent pregnancy. When combined with smoking, estrogen seems to especially pose a risk because smoking appears to increase the synthesis of thromboxane, which in turn activates platelets and increases constriction of arteries. Furthermore, smoking can cause direct vascular damage. In conjunction with the effects of estrogen on the coagulation system, smoking leads to a significantly higher risk of clot formation. The problem could be aggravated in the presence of underlying hypercoagulable tendency, which will likely contribute to higher risks of clotting in some patients.

74. What is CADASIL?

CADASIL is an acronym for Cerebral Autosomal Dominant Arteriopathy with Subcortical Infarcts and Leukoencephalopathy. This is an inherited neurological disease located on chromosome 19 that affect young individuals and is associated with migraine with aura, recurrent strokes, mood disorder and ultimately dementia. The mean age at onset of symptoms is 45 years, although the migraine symptoms occur a few years earlier. The migraines are often more severe and are accompanied by other neurological symptoms, including transient paralysis on one side of the body. The disease may go undiagnosed because the symptoms may overlap with other more common conditions and the family history may not always be clear. In some cases, CADASIL has been confused with multiple sclerosis because of clinical and imaging similarities. The cause of the disease is likely related to the deposit of abnormal proteins in the wall of the arteries, resulting in narrowing and ultimately blockage of the artery. There is no known treatment for this disorder. However, maximizing treatment for vascular disease is highly recommended because this can help limit additional damage to the artery from other more controllable factors.

PART ELEVEN

Medical Treatment of Ischemic Strokes

When do you give tissue plasminogen activator (t-PA)?

How are transient ischemic attacks treated?

What is the best blood-thinning medication to prevent stroke?

More . . .

Ischemic stroke is a stroke where the blood flow to a specific part of the brain is severely compromised to cause brain damage. The brain is extremely sensitive to decreased blood flow. The longer the blood is restricted, the less likely that the brain will recover, even if flow is reestablished. In general, the risk of ischemic stroke per week is approximately 1 in 5500 in patients aged 65 to 84 years. The risk of stroke increases to 1 in 2000 weekly for smokers. The overall risk of recurrence in persons who have had a stroke is twice as high as the risk of a first stroke. Depending on the etiologic mechanism of the stroke, the recurrence rate in individual patients varies from almost zero in some patients to 26% per 24 months in patients with symptomatic carotid artery stenosis and 12% per 12 months in those with nonvalvular atrial fibrillation.

The only approved treatment for acute stroke is the clot-busting drug tissue plasminogen activator (t-PA). Other treatments are given primarily to prevent a second stroke. However, acutely many other issues arise after a stroke as well that could impact recovery. In this section we discuss the use of t-PA, aspirin, clopidogrel, ticlopidine (Ticlid), Aggrenox, warfarin, and heparin.

75. When do you give tissue plasminogen activator (t-PA)?

Tissue plasminogen activator or t-PA is a clot-busting drug first introduced to treat heart attacks. Eventually, the National Institute of Neurological Disorders and Stroke (NINDS), sponsored a clinical trial testing its benefits in stroke, and the results were published in 1995. t-PA was found to be helpful in treating some strokes as long as the drug was given in the initial 3 hours after the onset of symptoms. Although patients with clear-cut symptoms of stroke and who present before the 3-hour window should receive t-PA, there are many confounding factors and controversy regarding the appropriate use of t-PA in some patients with ischemic stroke. One of the major misconceptions about the use of t-PA is the true benefit of this medication as reflected by the number of patients who have minimal to no residual deficits at 3 months. In evaluating the benefits of a treatment, we can use several statistical terms. The two most commonly used terms are "relative" and "absolute" differences. In the NINDS study the relative improvement in the treated group was approximately 30% but the absolute difference between the t-PA group and the placebo group was actually around 12% (i.e., 100 patients must be treated for 12 patients to have a positive response). Furthermore, since the publication of the NINDS study in 1995, many review articles have provided information regarding the type of strokes that benefit the most from t-PA and the type of stroke that are more likely to have bleeding complications after t-PA. Although the NINDS demonstrated a relatively better outcome in 30% (absolute difference was 12%) of patients, the greatest benefit from the NINDS trial was noted in lacunar strokes (small deep vessels) and a smaller benefit was noted in patients with cardioembolic strokes. The major risk of t-PA was hemorrhage, which was seen in 6%, half of which were fatal.

There have been several concerns in regards to the published NINDS results. One of the major concerns has been the relatively low numbers enrolled in this trial. For example, although the study screened thousands of patients, the NINDS study enrolled a total of 624 patients in the treatment and placebo groups. Another concern is that improvements in the lacunar stroke group were difficult to explain considering the known pathological nature of the disease. Finally, the cardioembolic group, the group that would potentially benefit the most, had the least dramatic improvement. Fast forward to now when physicians have had several years to test t-PA in the real world. Since 1995 there have been several studies evaluating the benefits of t-PA and most confirm these benefits. We also now know that t-PA is of limited benefit in large clots, such as the ones seen when the carotid artery is blocked or when one of its major branches, the middle cerebral artery, is blocked.

Medical Treatment of Ischemic Strokes

Therefore other techniques are being explored to help open blocked vessels. The application of clot-busting drugs directly into the clot could potentially eliminate some of the complications with intravenous administration of t-PA. Furthermore, injecting the clot-busting drug directly into the clot allows for mechanical disruption of the clot, which increases the drug's ability to dissolve the clot. As a result a trial was completed using intraarterial ProUK (a different clot-busting) to treat patients with large middle cerebral artery strokes (usually beyond 3 hours). Preliminary results were encouraging, but the U.S. Food and Drug Administration withheld approval of ProUK. Other techniques such as combining both intraarterial and intravenous t-PA have been explored.

Retrieval devices have also shown some promising results. The MERCI device is a corkscrew wire that is inserted in the clot and then pulled with retrieval of the clot and opening of the artery. Clinical outcome using this device is unknown at this time. These trials demonstrate the continuous search for better treatment for occluded large arteries. Since the NINDS trial established a certain "standard" of care for acute stroke, it has become difficult to introduce or test other treatments for strokes presenting within the first 3 hours, unless the proposed new treatment is combined with intravenous t-PA. Because t-PA only benefits some patients, research is needed to improve selection before treatment and to help find patients who could be nonresponders to t-PA but candidates for other treatment or candidates for enrollment in a clinical trial.

76. How are transient ischemic attacks treated?

The occurrence of a transient ischemic attack indicates transient interruption of blood supply to a certain region of the brain. Therefore the aim of treatment is to help reduce the risk of stroke. The physician should also investigate the cause of the symptoms to determine the best possible treatment. The first-line treatment for patients with transient ischemia is

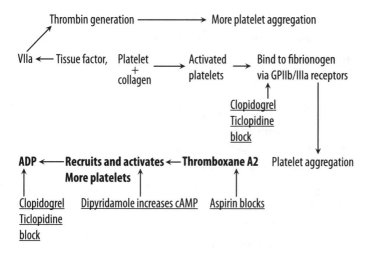

Figure 9   Factors that contribute to aggregation of platelets and oral drugs that influence platelet function (simplified)

aspirin. Aspirin is a drug that inhibits the binding of platelets; this in turn helps prevent a clot from forming and can also help reduce inflammation around the damaged artery. Data from several clinical studies have demonstrated the benefit of aspirin in reducing the risk of stroke in patients who have experienced a stroke or transient ischemic attack. Other antiplatelet agents are available, which may also be used either alone or in combination with aspirin. Figure 9 shows a simplified diagram of the role of platelets in the clotting system and drugs that influence the platelet function.

77. What is the best blood-thinning medication to prevent stroke?

There is no one specific medication that works for all types of strokes. There are generally two different types of medications: those that inhibit platelets and those that prevent a clot from forming. Platelets are part of the blood and serve an important function in stopping bleeding. However, platelets can also trigger the formation of clots on the inside of an artery. Therefore the logic behind using drugs that inhibit platelets is that by preventing the platelets from sticking to the inside of the artery, we can potentially prevent a bigger clot from forming. However, there are other ways that platelets can initiate a clot that have nothing to do with platelet aggregation.

Originally, aspirin was designed as a pain killer, but ultimately its ability to inhibit platelet aggregation was discovered. Acetylsalicylic acid, otherwise known as aspirin, irreversibly inhibits cyclooxygenase-1, which in turn reduces the activities of thromboxane A_2, which is necessary for platelet aggregation and for constriction of arteries. Because platelets do not have the ability to make more cyclooxygenase-1, small doses of aspirin inhibit platelet aggregation for the life of the platelet. By preventing platelet aggregation, the formation of a clot is hindered although not completely suppressed.

Although aspirin is an effective drug in inhibiting platelet function and in reducing the risk of strokes and heart attacks, there are several other drugs that can also inhibit platelets and reduce the risk of vascular events. However, none of the antiplatelet drugs we have now prevents 100% of ischemic strokes. The best that we can hope to achieve with these drugs is reduction in the risk of stroke by about 30%.

The reason that these antiplatelet drugs do not prevent all transient ischemic attacks or strokes is that transient ischemia can be caused by mechanisms other than traditional clots. Such mechanisms include reduced blood flow through an artery, a phenomenon that can occur in large and small arteries. Other causes for stroke include cholesterol emboli and other debris that may be in the wall of arteries leading to the brain. Although antithrombotic drugs may help prevent a clot from forming under some circumstances, the sequence of events that can lead to a stroke is far more complicated than simply the formation of a clot. Therefore antithrombotic drugs alone may not be "curative."

It is important to discern the cause of the transient ischemia to design the best treatment. For example, if symptoms were caused by a narrowed carotid artery, then treatment for the carotid artery needs to be implemented. If symptoms are originating from the heart, as may be the case in patients with atrial fibrillation, then treatment needs to be initiated with warfarin if deemed appropriate. In the long term, any potential risk factors that lead to the symptoms of transient ischemia also need to be controlled.

78. Are higher doses of aspirin more effective?

The dose of aspirin that can inhibit the aggregation of circulating platelets is approximately 100 mg, which can achieve its goal of inhibiting platelet aggregation in approximately 20 minutes. Smaller doses of aspirin accomplish the same goal but over a few days. A baby aspirin contains 81 mg of acetylsalicylic acid per tablet, whereas an adult aspirin contains 325 mg of acetylsalicylic acid. It has been suggested that based on the other known chemical effects that result in inhibition of prostacyclin, a protein produced by the lining of the arteries, there may be a paradoxical effect with the use of high doses of aspirin that can lead to platelet aggregation and constriction of arteries. However, these findings may not be clinically relevant because multiple clinical studies with doses of more than four adult-sized aspirin a day demonstrate similar statistical benefits to much smaller doses of aspirin.

79. What is the correct dose of aspirin to help prevent strokes?

There have been over 150 studies looking at the benefits of aspirin in patients with strokes and/or heart attacks. The dose of aspirin in these studies varied from 75 mg a day to as much as 1500 mg a day. The benefit seemed to be similar with any of the doses used. Overall, the studies demonstrated a reduction in heart attacks and strokes by approximately 22%. Another way to look at this is that aspirin prevented 36 vascular events per 1000 patients who had a previous stroke or transient ischemic attack and who were treated for a period slightly over 2 years. Therefore the recommendations so far are to take a maximum of 325 mg per day, but preferably less due to the paradoxical effects of clotting that theoretically can occur and also due to the potential of increasing the risk for bleeding from ulcers. The risk of developing a significant bleeding complication from higher dose aspirin can be twice as high as in patients treated with placebo. Although the risk for bleeding doubles, the number of patients who suffer from bleeding related to aspirin is very small, estimated to be 1.3 per 1000 patients.

80. Are there alternatives to aspirin?

A small number of patients develop either allergy or sensitivity to aspirin. Some of this sensitivity presents with gastrointestinal discomfort, breathing issues, or even bleeding from a gastric ulcer. Some patients may do well with a smaller dose of aspirin, but other alternatives exist to include clopidogrel and ticlopidine (Ticlid). Both medications act differently from aspirin in that they bind to a receptor that allows for platelet aggregation. Ticlopidine (Ticlid) is used infrequently because of the gastrointestinal side effects and the need for repeated blood tests during the first 3 months of therapy to monitor for a rare occurrence of precipitous drop in white blood cell count. Clopidogrel (Plavix) has fewer side effects but has been reported to infrequently cause a serious blood disorder known as thrombotic thrombocytopenic purpura.

81. Is clopidogrel or ticlopidine (Ticlid) as effective as aspirin in preventing stroke?

Ticlopidine has been studied extensively, and the evidence demonstrated significant benefit for ticlopidine over aspirin or placebo, with an overall risk reduction of 27%. Furthermore, the ticlopidine studies were able to demonstrate that women, African-Americans, those who had an event while on aspirin,

and patients who had transient ischemia or stroke in the vertebral basilar circulation benefited the most. Surprisingly, the
benefits for clopidogrel in stroke have been less impressive.
Much of the data regarding clopidogrel and stroke come from
the CAPRIE study published in 1996. The CAPRIE study
enrolled patients who had a recent stroke, myocardial infarction, or symptomatic disease in the peripheral arteries. The
study compared the benefits of clopidogrel to an adult aspirin.
Although there was an overall reduction of stroke, heart attacks, or vascular death by 8.7%, the benefit for patients who
suffered from only a stroke seemed to be insignificant. It has
been calculated that treatment with clopidogrel prevents one
recurrent stroke for each 125 patients treated, whereas treatment with ticlopidine (Ticlid) prevents one recurrent stroke
for each 40 patients treated. Other studies have suggested
that perhaps there is a benefit to combining clopidogrel and
aspirin; however, a recent study demonstrated that the combination of these drugs exposes the patient to a very high
risk of bleeding. The combination of aspirin and clopidogrel
is frequently used after stenting of the vessels in the heart,
although the risks of bleeding make this combination risky in
patients with recent strokes or transient ischemic attacks.

82. How effective is dipyridamole?

This medication affects platelet function by several mechanisms independent of effects on cyclooxygenase-1 (i.e., different from aspirin or clopidogrel). Unlike aspirin or clopidogrel,
the effects on platelet function are short lived. Because dipyridamole affects platelet function through a different mechanism and is relatively cheap, in the past and without significant
scientific evidence, many physicians used it in combination
with aspirin to further decrease platelet aggregation. More
recently, clinical studies demonstrated the benefit of combination therapy. A small dose of aspirin at 25 mg combined with
200 mg of dipyridamole in a slow release capsule (Aggrenox)
given twice a day is more beneficial than either dipyridamole
or aspirin alone. With the use of Aggrenox, the risk of stroke

was decreased by 37% compared with approximately 17% with either aspirin or dipyridamole. It has been calculated that treatment with Aggrenox prevents one recurrent stroke for every 33 patients treated. The side effects of dipyridamole include headaches, dizziness, and diarrhea. In the clinical trials approximately 6% of patients dropped out of the study because of headaches. The headaches usually occur at the beginning of treatment and can be minimized by initiation of treatment with one capsule a day for approximately a week before increasing the medication to the recommended dose of one capsule twice a day. Some physicians have criticized the outcome of this trial because it was focused on stroke and not other vascular events, which may be equally as important as stroke. Although generally it appears that the combination treatment of aspirin and dipyridamole is more effective in reducing stroke, heart attacks, or sudden death than aspirin alone, many cardiologists prefer the use of clopidogrel, sometimes in combination with aspirin.

83. Can I continue to take aspirin and ibuprofen for my joint pain?

Individuals taking ibuprofen or other medications like it, such as naproxen, do not generally consult with their physician before taking what is deceptively considered benign treatment for pain. Studies have convincingly demonstrated that the administration of ibuprofen or naproxen with aspirin undermines the ability of aspirin to inhibit cyclooxygenase-1 in the platelets; consequently, the ability of aspirin to inhibit platelet aggregation is significantly diminished. Therefore combining ibuprofen with aspirin significantly hinders the antiplatelet activities of aspirin, and as a result aspirin will not prevent clot formation, increasing the risk of strokes and heart attacks. Taking ibuprofen at approximately 600 mg three times per day results in significant reduction in preventing platelet aggregation within 24 hours. Taking aspirin several hours before ibuprofen helps mitigate this adverse interaction. Other drugs that have different pharmacological action on the platelets, such as clopidogrel or ticlopidine (Ticlid), theoretically also mitigate the effects of ibuprofen-like medications.

84. Is the discontinuation of aspirin for elective surgery necessary?

The use of antiplatelet agents in patients with cerebrovascular disease reduces the risk of secondary stroke, myocardial infarction (heart attack), and vascular death by 22%. Antiplatelet drugs have been shown to be effective for both short-term and long-term prevention of secondary ischemic stroke after transient ischemia or completed ischemic stroke. Discontinuation of low-dose aspirin use may lead to hazardous events, such as stroke, myocardial infarction, or even cardiovascular death, but the exact incidence of vascular events after aspirin cessation remains uncertain. The rate of any vascular event during long-term low-dose aspirin use is comparatively low at about 1.1 per 1000 patients per week. Withholding aspirin perioperatively for 7 days would add a risk of about 0.3 additional patients for every 1000 patients per week.

Management strategies using available literature are difficult to extrapolate on this subject due to variations in patient populations, procedures, antiplatelet regimen, definitions of events, and durations of follow-up. Randomized controlled trials are needed to provide reasonable estimates of the perioperative risk of thromboembolism and bleeding risks of continuation of therapy.

Literature on continuation of medically necessary aspirin before surgery is less influential; however, reports in ophthalmological and urological journals suggest that continuation of aspirin is rational and without undue hemorrhagic risks. Although controversial, continuation of aspirin has been recommended in patients undergoing urgent coronary artery bypass. Moreover, a course of antiplatelet therapy should be completed after coronary stenting for a minimum of 6 weeks to reduce the frequency of stent thrombosis and other adverse events. Clotting of the stents can occur shortly after interruption of antiplatelet therapy.

In summary, discontinuation of antiplatelet agent(s) should be conducted on a case-by-case basis. Under most circumstances, antiplatelet agents can safely be continued before surgery in most patients. The decision to discontinue the aspirin or alternative antiplatelet medications should be considered if the patients' bleeding risk while on the medication exceeds the risk of a secondary thromboembolic event while off treatment transiently. Furthermore, patients considered at high risk for recurring vascular events after discontinuation of antiplatelet therapy are those with a history of transient ischemic attack or stroke within 2 years and patients who have undergone recent percutaneous coronary intervention.

85. When is warfarin used to prevent strokes?

One other drug that is frequently used to help prevent ischemic strokes is warfarin (Coumadin). This is a pill taken to "thin" the blood. This medication does not literally thin the blood but helps prevent red clots from forming by inhibiting vitamin K, which is essential for proclotting factors. The only scientific evidence for its utility is in patients who have atrial fibrillation. In atrial fibrillation the irregular heart beat together with inefficient contractions of the heart chambers promotes clots to form inside the heart. These clots then can travel to the brain as well as to other organs. Multiple scientific studies (see p 24, question 16) have shown that warfarin (Coumadin) is beneficial in reducing the risk of stroke in patients with atrial fibrillation.

From the perspective of clinical experience, warfarin is a difficult drug to use and requires close follow-up to prevent major changes in the required levels of "thinning." The effectiveness of warfarin (Coumadin) is measured by a blood test referred to as the INR (International Normalization Ratio, see Glossary). Under most circumstance the recommended INR is between 2 and 3. The higher the number, the "thinner the blood." INR levels above 3 increase the risk of bleeding, and INR levels below 2 appear to be less effective. This narrow safe and therapeutic range makes management of patients on warfarin difficult and sometimes unpredictable. Because of the unpredictability of treatment with warfarin and individual responses to specific doses, when warfarin is initiated the INR should be tested at least once a week and then when stable, once a month.

Several stratification schemes have been proposed to help physicians decide on the risk and benefits of anticoagulation with warfarin for patients with atrial fibrillation. The most useful is the CHADS2 criteria (Cardiac Failure, Hypertension, Age, Diabetes, Stroke). Two points are assigned for a history of stroke or transient ischemic attack and 1 point each is assigned for age over 75 years, a history of hypertension, diabetes, or recent heart failure. According to this scheme, patients with low scores had a risk of 1.5% per year, those with medium scores had a risk of 3.3%, and those with high scores had a risk of stroke of almost 6% per year. Warfarin is associated with a risk for bleeding that should be weighted against the benefits. In patients aged 60 years and younger with no other risk factors, the risk of stroke from atrial fibrillation is very small and anticoagulation may not be warranted. Many patients may not tolerate the recommended levels of anticoagulation as measured by INR. The recommended INR for effective and safe anticoagulation is between 2.0 and 3.0. However, if patients seem to have some bleeding complication, options may include the use of lower intensity anticoagulation with INR between 1.6 and 2.5. Studies have demonstrated that the risk of bleeding in the brain occurs in approximately 0.3% to 2% of patients on warfarin. The highest risk of bleeding occurs in patients older than 80 years old or in those with history of transient ischemic attack, stroke, congestive heart failure, diabetes, high blood pressure, and heart attack and in patients with INR greater than 3.

Another major indication for the use of warfarin is metallic heart valve. Under those circumstance the level of anticoagulation is higher than that in atrial fibrillation and sometimes, if there is evidence of recurring stroke despite the use of warfarin, aspirin is added to warfarin. Another common use of warfarin is in the prevention of stroke in patients with a floppy left ventricle, although no evidence of its benefits exists yet. Warfarin in combination with aspirin has been used to prevent blockage of coronary arteries and peripheral arteries after treatment. Warfarin is used for myriad of other conditions with little to no scientific evidence for such use. Like in many other fields of medicine, medical treatment for each patient needs to be tailored to fit that specific condition. Scientific information and recommendations from professional organizations provide a guide to treatment for a typical patient. Many patients have strokes that do not fit profiles of recent scientific studies.

Several studies have shown that it is difficult to maintain the INR in the appropriate range even when the blood is tested frequently. Some studies have shown that the INR may not be in the correct range in about 40% of the measurements. The difficulties in monitoring and maintaining effects of warfarin in a safe and effective range has prompted pharmaceutical companies to test other products that may be easier to use and monitor. Unfortunately, so far no other alternatives to warfarin exist. A drug that was recently investigated, Ximelagatran, showed benefits equal to warfarin in preventing strokes with fewer hemorrhages. However, this drug was not approved because of concerns regarding liver toxicity.

There have been studies to test the utility of warfarin in other types of strokes, including those from high-grade narrowing of arteries inside the head (WASID trial) and in patients who had recurring stroke or transient ischemia from factors other than operable vascular problem or atrial fibrillation (WARSS trial). Both studies demonstrated no benefits to warfarin over aspirin in prevention of another stroke, yet patients had a higher rate of hemorrhages with warfarin. However, as with other clinical studies there have been criticisms regarding both studies.

86. What should I do if I notice an excessive amount of bleeding while I am on warfarin?

Warfarin is a drug that if not closely monitored can cause significant bleeding complication. Unfortunately, many patients are not as compliant with the medication as they should be, with many patients skipping doses of warfarin without notifying the physician. Also, many do not follow the strict dietary guidelines or they take over-the-counter medications that interact with warfarin, such as acetaminophen (Tylenol). Physicians also are sometimes unaware of the interactions of seemingly routine medications such as antibiotics. As a result patients' INR level can dramatically fluctuate. High INR over 3.0 can increase the risk of bleeding. If bleeding is noted you should contact your primary care physician immediately or go to the emergency room. Blood tests or adjustments to the dose of warfarin need to be done. If excessive bleeding results in symptoms or a decrease in the level of hematocrit, then reversing the effects of warfarin and transfusion of red blood cells may be necessary.

87. Is it necessary to discontinue warfarin for minor surgeries and dental cleaning?

Current recommendations are to continue anticoagulation during certain surgical procedures based on both lack of increased hemorrhagic complications and the potential of thrombotic events on discontinuation. Dental procedures, including prosthetics, endodontics, restorations, extractions, and hygiene, are among the procedures for which recommendations have been made to continue anticoagulant therapy during the perioperative period to avoid thromboembolic complications. Ophthalmic procedures, including cataract surgery, can be performed successfully in patients who continue taking warfarin. Even in more invasive procedures such as transurethral prostatectomy and cardiac surgery, continuation of warfarin has been recommended. The discontinuation of warfarin should be weighted carefully against the possibility of stroke and risk of bleeding complication from the procedure. The general guidelines available from professional organizations suggest that in low-risk patients for recurrent stroke, it is reasonable to discontinue anticoagulation for no more than 1 week. In high-risk patients some level of anticoagulation should be maintained, usually with low-molecular-weight heparin. Many physicians and dentists are not comfortable continuing warfarin while performing certain procedures. Each procedure has potential risks, and therefore there is no general recommendation to cover all procedures and all patients. When in doubt, maintaining some anticoagulation is better than discontinuing it if the risk of bleeding is acceptable or if local measures to control bleeding are effective.

88. What happens if I don't take warfarin for a few days?

As discussed earlier, warfarin is a medication that can be difficult to manage because of the "nuisance" factor. Some studies have suggested that up to 30% of patients are not compliant with either taking the warfarin as recommended or do not obtain the recommended blood test. Stopping warfarin for a few days results in loss of the effects of warfarin. If it is absolutely necessary to stop warfarin, then it is best to stop it for the shortest period possible and restart it as soon as possible. Reports suggest a "rebound" phenomenon with an increased tendency for clotting after the discontinuation of warfarin due to an increase in levels of activated factor VII, prothrombin fragments, and D-dimers. Although the clinical significance of this rebound phenomenon for stroke is not entirely clear yet, elevation in these factors has been documented in patients who later develop clots in the deep veins (deep venous thrombosis) after hip surgery and also in patients with recurrence of deep venous thrombosis. Discontinuation of warfarin in preparation for surgery can result in increased risk for stroke: In one study the discontinuation of warfarin accounted for approximately 7% of all the embolic strokes in a 12-month period. The strokes occurred on the average 5 days after the discontinuation of warfarin.

89. Is heparin used to treat strokes?

Heparin, and other heparin-like drugs, is used more ubiquitously in cardiology and whenever interventional procedures are performed on arteries with catheters and stents. When heparin is used, its effects on the clotting system are measured by a test called activated partial thromboplastin time. The amount of heparin and its effects on the clotting system are not always predictable. Heparin can be given intravenously or subcutaneously (under the skin). Its use in stroke is empirical, often done with good intentions but without scientific foundation. Some physicians believe that heparin can prevent further clot formation in a much narrowed symptomatic artery or that heparin can prevent further progression of symptoms after a stroke. Accumulating evidence over the years has made heparin a less attractive drug for the treatment of ischemic stroke. So far there are no data to suggest that heparin is better than aspirin after a transient ischemic attack or stroke.

Early studies on the benefits and complication of heparin suggested a relatively high risk for bleeding after a stroke, at approximately 24%. The occurrence of bleeding seemed to depend on the level of anticoagulation (i.e., the higher the activated partial thromboplastin time, the more likely the bleed). Other investigators, who retrospectively reviewed outcome in patients receiving heparin, suggested that patients who were not receiving adequate amounts of heparin had a risk for having another stroke. Because of the confusing and nonscientific information that was available, a task force was formed to review the evidence and make recommendations. The Cerebral Embolism Task Force published their recommendation in 1989. It was concluded that recurrence of embolic stroke in the first 2 weeks was low, and bleeding complications were more common in patients with large stroke and those with high levels of anticoagulation and early bleeding changes on CT of the brain. The task force recommended delay of anti-coagulation for at least 48 hours. In a large clinical study, the 1997 International Stroke Trial, over 19,000 patients were randomized to receive either aspirin or heparin. This study demonstrated that the risk for another stroke in the first 2 weeks after stroke was 2.9% in the heparin group and 3.8% in the aspirin group. The bleeding complication was significant for the heparin group at approximately 1.2%; the bleeding complication was 0.9% for those taking aspirin and 0.4% in patients who received no treatment. The conclusion of this study was that although there may be a marginal benefit to heparin, the bleeding complications erased any of those benefits. Although there are many critics of this study, it remains the only study that provided some idea of the risk of recurrence and risk of bleeding as well as benefits to heparin and aspirin in acute stroke.

Other studies have used synthetic forms of heparin, known as heparinoid. The TOAST study published in 1993 demonstrated no overall benefit to strokes and no evidence that this type of heparin helps prevent the progression of stroke. As with any study, however, investigators have looked at subgroups that could benefit; as a result, benefit was suggested in those with disease of the large arteries, such as carotid arteries, and in those with embolic strokes originating from the heart. However, the value of subgroup analysis is questioned because the design of the study was not formatted in such a way to allow for this type of statistical analysis. Another form of heparin, known as low-molecular-weight heparin, was evaluated for its potential for stroke benefit. Here again no apparent short-term benefit was seen, although in those patients receiving low-molecular-weight heparin there was overall fewer patients with poor outcome at 6 months.

As a result of the above review, it appears that the use of heparin under most circumstances is not indicated in the acute treatment of stroke. The use of heparin during neurointerventional procedures may be necessary to prevent clot formation with catheter use. The use of heparin for high-grade symptomatic narrowing or dissections of arteries may be justifiable but is without scientific merit. Aspirin and other aspirin-like compounds are not a cure for stroke either, but we know that aspirin can help in preventing a subsequent stroke.

Medical Treatment of Ischemic Strokes

PART TWELVE

Complications from Stroke

What are the most common
complications from stroke?

How should blood pressure be managed
in an acute stroke?

More . . .

During the acute phase of a stroke many potential complications can occur and can result in significant morbidity and mortality. Factors that increase the chances for a bad outcome include prior strokes, multiple strokes or transient ischemic attacks, older age, peripheral vascular disease, enlarged heart, abnormal heart valves, atrial fibrillation, elevated blood sugar, fevers, swelling in the brain, aspiration pneumonia and other infections, and pulmonary emboli. Once the patient is admitted to the hospital after an acute stroke, most of the subsequent care is aimed at controlling and limiting the potential of complications. The job of the medical team is truly to put out fires that can spring up at any time during hospitalization and rehabilitation. The body has a remarkable ability to recover, but acutely when the body is under stress with decreased mobility and limited nutrition, the body's internal system can become chaotic. The impact of the stroke also goes beyond local damage to the brain. Many brain structures are critical for the function of vital organs and in regulating the immune system as well as levels of hormones. Therefore damage to the brain from a stroke has adverse diffuse effects on the body that can hinder recovery.

90. What are the most common complications from stroke?

A patient's neurological condition can worsen after a stroke as a result of multiple complications, including seizures, extension of the stroke, swelling of the damaged area, bleeding in an ischemic stroke or additional bleeding in hemorrhagic stroke, congestive heart failure, other heart disease, gastrointestinal bleeding, urinary tract infection, deep venous thrombosis (clots in leg veins), pneumonia, pulmonary embolus (clots in the lungs), malnutrition, and seizures. Complications in the first 3 days are due to changes in the brain from the stroke; this occurs in approximately 30% of patients. Later complications, between 3 and 7 days, are associated with non-neurological complications, such as infections.

Seizures in stroke: Despite multiple recent studies, the exact incidence and the risks leading to seizures are still not well defined. Some studies have suggested that prevalence of seizures in stroke patients is around 4%, with most seizures occurring in patients who suffered from ischemic stroke. Other studies have found significantly higher rates of seizures, around 9%, with the highest risk in patients with hemorrhagic strokes. The major risk factor for seizure is the location in the cortex (superficial part of the brain). Most seizures occur in the acute phase after a stroke. In some long-term studies, approximately 2.5% to 9% of patients with stroke had recurrence of seizure. Recurrence was highest in patients with early onset of seizures and in those with large strokes. Treatment for seizures should be initiated after the first seizure, because seizure recurrence significantly impacts recovery. Sometimes the seizures are obvious, but other times seizures can be difficult to recognize, because the symptoms may be subtle. Sometimes the simple fact that the patient with a stroke appears to have more neurological deficits than can be accounted for by the location and the size of the stroke may trigger additional investigations for seizures as well as other factors such as infections. There are multiple medications that can be used to control seizures. The new generation drugs have fewer side effects. It is not clear if one specific drug has an advantage over another. In selecting a medication to treat seizures, one has to consider the potential side effects, interactions with other medications, and impact on rehabilitation.

Pulmonary embolus: Pulmonary embolus (PE) refers to a clot that travels from a vein and blocks blood circulation in the lungs. If the pulmonary embolus is small it can be asymptomatic, but a large pulmonary embolus can result in death due to poor oxygen exchange. Pulmonary embolus has been reported to occur in approximately 1% of patients who suffer from stroke and to account for 25% of deaths, especially during the first 4 weeks after a stroke. The major cause for PE is a clot in the veins, called deep venous thrombosis (DVT).

Symptomatic pulmonary embolus is treated with clot-busting drugs, heparin, or mechanical retrieval of the clot.

Deep venous thrombosis after a stroke: Deep venous thrombosis (DVT) is very common after a stroke and results in paralysis of the leg. The estimated incidence of DVT in stroke population is approximately 50% in the first 2 weeks after a stroke. The clot occurs usually in the immobile leg and usually within the first week after the stroke. Additional patients with DVT are diagnosed during the rehabilitation period. The Post-Stroke Rehabilitation Outcomes Project (2005) demonstrated that nearly an additional 6% of patients develop DVT during the rehabilitation period. Because this is a relatively frequent occurrence in patients with a paralyzed leg and in patients who are generally bedridden, health care professionals are aware of the need to monitor for any swelling or discomfort in the limb, which then may lead to the diagnosis of DVT. Unfortunately, many patients with DVT do not develop any obvious signs or symptoms that can help alert the physicians. Therefore all patients with the potential of developing DVT should be treated with preventative measures and then when necessary be screened for DVT, because preventative measures are not successful all of the time.

A recent study with enoxaparin (Lovenox), a form of low-molecular-weight heparin, demonstrated greater benefit of this drug over regular heparin by reducing the risk of DVT by 43%. However, this and other studies have demonstrated that despite treatment with blood-thinning medications, venous clots can still occur in 8% to 18% of patients, depending on the drug being used. Therefore, although blood-thinning medications are helpful, mobility is a critical element in preventing this complication. The use of compression (pneumatic) boots in addition to the blood-thinning medication is desirable. Compression boots alone are not as effective as the blood-thinning medication alone or when blood-thinning medication is combined with compression boots. There are circumstances when the use of blood-thinning medications is not safe such as may occur acutely after an intracerebral hemorrhage; therefore the only short-term treatment to help prevent DVT is to use pneumatic boots. Once a DVT is discovered, patients who do not have any contraindication to blood-thinning medication are placed initially on heparin and then are converted to warfarin. Patients sometimes continue taking warfarin for more than 6 months depending on the risk factors that can lead to recurrence of venous clots. In patients who cannot be placed on blood-thinning medications, the management then requires the placement of a filter in the inferior vena cava, a large vein in the abdomen, and the chest. The filter prevents significant blood clots from reaching the lungs.

Swelling in the brain: All strokes cause some local swelling, but larger strokes and strokes in specific areas of the brain are more likely to cause further complications and hinder recovery. Large strokes affecting the middle cerebral artery territory is one of the most devastating strokes because it usually affects almost half of the hemisphere. The large size of the stroke, the leakage of fluids, and inflammation all contribute to potentially more damage to the surrounding normal brain. A large stroke in the middle cerebral artery territory with swelling, often referred to as "malignant" middle cerebral artery infarct, is associated with 80% mortality. Another part of the brain that can be associated with devastating outcome with excessive swelling is in the cerebellum. Because of the location of the cerebellum, in a fairly tight compartment near the brainstem and near the fourth ventricle, the swelling can be fatal. The swelling can compress normal brain and can result in additional damage to the brain as a result of compromised blood flow or by causing small hemorrhages from tarring of blood vessels within the brain.

Treatment of swelling in the brain: Not all swelling requires treatment. Early swelling in a large stroke as evident on CT may imply that the worse is still to come. Swelling peaks around 3 to 4 days after stroke. During that period close monitoring of the patient for changes in neurological function is critical. If the swelling appears to be affecting neurological function, then measures must be taken to help minimize the effect of the swelling on adjacent viable brain. Restriction of certain types of fluids and the use of diuretics (drugs that eliminate excess water) are reasonable early first steps. However, this strategy is temporary, because the excess free water can only be eliminated from normal brain tissue and not the damaged brain. Hyperventilation is another temporary strategy. Under those circumstances the patient is intubated and the ventilation rate is set higher than usual. Hyperventilation eliminates the carbon dioxide, resulting in limited constriction of vessels that in turn helps decrease the swelling. Hyperventilation is very temporary and may adversely affect the brain with its vasoconstrictive effects. Vasoconstriction implies decreased blood flow to the brain. Although that may be tolerated in a normal brain, a brain with recent stroke has parts that are precariously positioned in a zone with decreased blood flow but not dead. These areas of the brain, known as the "penumbra," are potentially salvageable and therefore even slight compromise of circulation may result in cell death. Steroids to decrease swelling have been studied in a variety of different types of strokes, but no benefit was ever demonstrated with apparently increased level of infectious complication. Sedation with barbiturate medication has been suggested as an alternative treatment to lower pressure inside the head from the excessive swelling. Barbiturate also results in suppression of electrical signal in the brain, which can help limit the damage in the area of the stroke. The major potential complication from the use of barbiturate is lowering of blood pressure, which is not desirable in an acute stroke.

In patients who develop significant and rapid swelling, surgery may be considered to help relieve the pressure. There are two situations where surgery is considered. The first is when a patient develops early swelling in a large portion of the brain after a stroke in the territory of the middle cerebral artery, often referred to as "malignant middle cerebral artery stroke." The other circumstance is when a large stroke affecting the cerebellum (near the brainstem) swells and begins to obstruct flow to the spinal fluid. A recent review of pooled data from three clinical studies looking at the benefit of surgery in improving outcome suggested that more patients had a favorable outcome and more patients survived with surgery than without surgery. The decision to proceed with decompressive surgery is not as simple as one would like. In one study, some patients who were surveyed after the procedure regretted their decision to pursue such a procedure. This is an important glimpse into the complex interactions between the level of disability and the quality of life of patients with such a large stroke. All the available studies show that patients older than 50 years generally did not fair well after these decompressive surgeries; therefore the surgery is best performed under the right circumstances in younger patients and only after lengthy discussions with the family regarding expectations of recovery.

Aspiration pneumonia: Under normal circumstances fluid and food are kept away from the windpipe (trachea) by a complex swallowing reflex. However, with strokes, many patients lose the ability to maintain normal swallowing reflexes, allowing for oral contents to drop in the trachea and then into the lungs. Because the oral–pharyngeal area is full of bacteria, the oral contents contaminate the more sterile environment of the lungs, causing infection and inflammation. Pneumonia is estimated to occur in 13% of patients with ischemic stroke and accounts for fivefold increased odds of death after a stroke. Because aspiration pneumonia is related to failure of swallowing mechanisms, early identification of patients at risk should help prevent aspiration pneumonia. Studies have shown that more severe strokes and older age increase the risk of aspiration. On the average, approximately half the patients admitted with stroke have difficulties swallowing (dysphagia). Therefore it is recommended that evaluation of swallowing on all patients with stroke should be done at the time of admission to the hospital and before initiating any oral intake. Studies have demonstrated that the implementation of protective measures against aspiration can be effective in decreasing the risk of aspiration pneumonia by 50% or more. The measures include maintaining the head of the bed at an angle greater than 45 degrees, not giving anything by mouth until the swallowing reflexes improve or recover, and, when appropriate, change the consistency of the food and use the chin-tuck technique. The good news is that more than half of the patients recover within a week and more recover at 1 month. The challenge for the future is to find ways to prevent most aspirations, because current measures are not completely effective.

Recurrence of stroke: Clinical or symptomatic recurrence of stroke in the first few days to 2 weeks after a stroke is considered low. The International Stroke Trial demonstrated that the recurrence is approximately 3% at 2 weeks. However, because of limitation of imaging in this trial, it is possible that these numbers are an underestimate of overall stroke recurrence. Other studies have suggested recurrence rates in the first month, 1 year, and 5 years to average 5%, 7%, and 30%, respectively. Using MRI, especially the "diffusion" sequence (see page 4), a recent study demonstrated that some patients, approximately 17%, may experience multiple strokes over a period of a few weeks before they present with the index event. Furthermore, patients who have evidence of multiple strokes of varying ages on the initial diffusion MRI or cardio-embolic source (clots from the heart) for their stroke were at an almost sevenfold and threefold increased risk, respectively, of having additional strokes at 30 days. Therefore the available evidence suggests that clinical recurrence appears to be low, but imaging studies suggest a substantially higher recurrence rate. It is not entirely clear at this time how the presence of silent strokes on MRI changes the management of patients acutely or subsequent to the initial stroke, but these data sug-

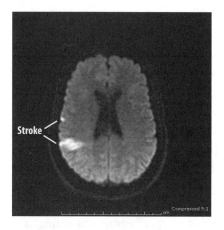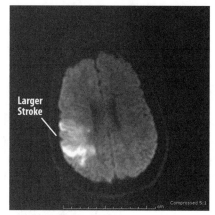

Figure 10   Diffusion MRIs. The scan on the left shows size of damage a few hours after stroke. The scan on the right shows the size of damage 24 hours after stroke.

gest that the risk of recurrence is higher than initially thought. The recurrence of strokes also is considered a significant factor in poor outcome after the initial stroke. Figure 10 shows expansion of stroke as seen on diffusion MRI.

Hemorrhagic transformation: Hemorrhagic transformation is when an ischemic stroke turns into a hemorrhagic stroke. This implies that there are changes within the area of stroke that allows for leakage of blood from damaged arteries. Not all hemorrhagic transformations cause additional damage to the brain; in fact, most hemorrhagic transformation results in punctate bleeds, causing no additional brain damage. Embolic strokes have the highest degree of hemorrhagic transformation. Some detailed studies of this condition using CT and cerebral angiography suggest that approximately 40% of ischemic strokes evolve into hemorrhagic stroke, although more than half were punctate hemorrhages, 11% developed massive bleeding, and 14% developed a small amount of bleeding. The mechanism of hemorrhagic transformation was initially thought to be related to reperfusion of damaged brain (i.e., reestablishing relatively high volume flow into areas of the brain with damaged arteries). However, other explanations

141

have also been proposed, such as enhanced blood flow from collaterals into the ischemic area, perhaps in conjunction with elevation in blood pressure, beyond the capabilities of the damaged brain to accommodate this flow.

Fevers in an acute stroke: Fever may occur due to infections, but if infections have been ruled out then the elevated body temperature (hyperthermia) is referred to as a "central fever." This is a common and spontaneous response in patients with stroke. Hyperthermia higher than 99.5°F in the first 24 hours is a predictor of poor outcome in stroke. There is usually a cascade of events that leads to hyperthermia, including cellular injury, abnormal activation of neurons, and liberation of toxic proteins such as cytokines, tumor necrosis factor-alpha, interleukin-1beta, and interleukin 6. As the stroke progresses and the clot disintegrates, flow is reestablished to the affected tissue. As a result, certain genes that promote inflammation become activated, making more proteins that are toxic to nearby cells increasing the amount of damage to the brain. This destructive cascade also promotes adhesion of white blood cells to the lining of the arteries (endothelium), encourages platelet aggregation, and therefore increases local clotting. Although these changes may not change the amount of cellular damage at the nidus of the stroke, there are usually areas nearby, the penumbra, that are "stunned" but not dead. With elevated temperature, there is an increase in the amount of production of substances that increase cellular injury. The energy requirement of the cell in this revved up environment is increased and the fuel of the cell, known as ATP, may get depleted quickly. When the cell runs out of fuel, it no longer is able to clear the toxins. All the evidence is consistent with the fact that hyperthermia is associated with poor outcome and may be deleterious to recovery from stroke. Animal studies have demonstrated the benefits of lowering body temperature in limiting the size of stroke, but human studies are still in their infancy. The recommendation, however, is to use medications to lower the body temperature at least until more evidence is available that demonstrates the benefits of more aggressive cooling.

Elevated blood sugar and stroke outcome: It is common to see an elevation in blood sugar during the acute phase of a stroke. Approximately 35% of patients with stroke have elevated blood sugar, but only half are known diabetics. In a normal individual, blood sugar is tightly controlled between 65 and 100 mg/dL. Elevated blood sugar in the setting of stroke is associated with increased short- and long-term mortality as well as increased cost. Hemorrhagic strokes and brainstem strokes have more severe elevation in blood sugar. It was commonly accepted that moderate levels of elevation in blood sugar in critically ill patients was beneficial for some organs, such as the brain, that rely on glucose for their energy supply. In fact, until 2002 it was acceptable to have blood sugar of 220 mg/dL in critically ill patients. During hypoxia (decreased oxygen supply), the brain, unlike other organs, decreases glucose uptake. Although this may appear to be contraintuitive to normal function of a stressed brain, in fact this is an important survival mechanism. When there is a decrease in oxygen supply, glucose use results in the accumulation of toxic lactic acid. Animal experiments have demonstrated a direct relationship between lactic acid levels and the degree of cellular injury as well as recovery. There is also an interesting paradox that occurs in areas of the brain that have partial flow after a stroke. Under those circumstances partial flow delivers glucose to areas of the brain with cellular injury and decreased overall blood supply; this leads to an increase in the levels of lactic acid. Elevation of blood sugar in acute stroke may be simply a reflection of occult diabetes, reaction to acute stress, or dysfunction of certain parts of the brain that regulate sugar. Similar to the effects of fever on the penumbra, which is the area that is stunned but not dead, elevated blood sugar results in irreversible damage in areas that are potentially salvageable.

Complications From Stroke

Patients with diabetes have an almost twofold increased risk of death after an acute heart attack. In patients with stroke, adverse outcomes were related to on-admission elevation of blood sugar. The elevation in blood sugar that correlated with worse outcome in stroke was surprisingly not excessively high, with evidence suggesting that poor outcome correlated with elevation just above 150 mg/dL. Similarly, patients who had elevated blood sugar who received the clot-busting drug tissue plasminogen activator (t-PA) for an acute stroke did poorly compared with those with normal blood sugar. Finally, elevated blood sugar was associated with larger size of stroke and reduced ability to salvage the penumbra. Studies have demonstrated that aggressive management of elevated blood sugar in patients with heart attack or patients in the surgical intensive care unit reduced mortality by 40%. Unfortunately, at least two large clinical studies in patients with stroke have not demonstrated any benefits to aggressive control of elevated blood sugar in patients with an acute stroke. However, one has to wonder if it is simply the elevated blood sugar that is the sole contributor to poor outcome. Logically, one would presume that correction of this problem should improve outcome. However, hypoxia (decreased level of oxygen supply) and elevated blood sugar may cause worsening through other mechanisms that are not rapidly reversible by normalizing blood sugar levels, such as changes within the cells at the molecular level and initiating the release of cellular factors that augment inflammation. Furthermore, animal models that seem to predict better outcome when elevated blood sugar is controlled have limited applicability to human brain. Nevertheless, the American College of Endocrinology Consensus Development Conference on Inpatient Diabetes and Metabolic Control recommend blood sugar levels of 110 mg/dL for patients in the intensive care unit and 110 to 180 mg/dL for noncritical patients. The tighter control of blood sugar may not directly influence areas of the brain with the stroke but can nevertheless help with the acute recovery by limiting the potential of metabolic changes related to elevated blood sugar and limit the risk of infection, which is more common when the blood sugar is elevated.

Aside from the physical and cognitive impairment, I suffer from fatigue. Not only do I require more sleep than I ever did pre-stroke, I also take two- to three-hour naps daily. I have had other complications too, specifically with my menstrual cycle, with severe hemorrhaging during my menstrual period. It was like a dam had been breached. I never understood whether this was due to the damage to my brain or the number of medicines I was ingesting. I had a D&C to help alleviate the bleeding. I also cannot regulate the temperature on my left side. Although the temperature of my limbs seems normal to the touch, my brain transmits the sensation that my limbs as burning with heat or freezing with cold.

91. How should blood pressure be managed in an acute stroke?

The answer is gingerly. However, to answer this properly, one must understand some of the basic issues related to the regulation of blood pressure and other concerns that impact management in acute stroke. Under normal conditions, blood flow to the vital organs remains constant in the face of changes in perfusion. This element of blood pressure control is known as "autoregulation" and is controlled by changes in the caliber of the small arteries. Autoregulation is rapid and complete within 15 to 30 seconds. Perfusion can fall by about 30% before blood flow inside the brain falls. In the presence of narrowed arteries, the autoregulatory reserve is diminished (i.e., drops in blood pressure are difficult to accommodate). The mechanism is not fully understood but requires intact and normally functioning arteries. Evidence from some clinical trials suggests that lowering the blood pressure in an acute stroke results in worsening the outcome in a subgroup of patients after a stroke (INWEST, 2003). Retrospective analysis of data from clinical trials such as the TOAST trial demonstrated better neurological outcome in patients with systolic blood pressure between 140 and 220 mm Hg and diastolic blood pressure between 70 and 110 mm Hg. A prospective review of variables contributing to worse outcome after acute stroke concluded that there was nearly a twofold risk of poor outcome with each 10% decrease in systolic blood pressure. Small studies published between 1997 and 2001 suggested that artificially raising blood pressure for a few days in acute stroke can be beneficial. These studies also suggested a threshold for the blood pressure that seems to help improve outcome. The threshold has been estimated at systolic blood pressure of 156 mm Hg. Although there is a fear that such treatment could increase the risk of heart attacks or intracerebral hemorrhage and may increase the degree of brain swelling after a stroke, available studies did not demonstrate an increase in complications or morbidity in those patients whose blood pressure was artificially increased. Furthermore, some of these small studies suggest that the benefit derived from induced hypertension in the acute stroke is sustainable when the blood pressure is allowed to drift to "normal" levels. The setting of an acute stroke is different from long-term need for the treatment of hypertension. Hypertension is a leading cause of strokes, and aggressive management of that condition for primary and secondary prevention is essential. Therefore lowering the blood pressure after the initial phase of an acute stroke is paramount in the overall management of risk factors for stroke.

PART THIRTEEN

Cardiac Arrest and Brain Injury

How can you determine recovery of brain
function after cardiac arrest?

More . . .

Approximately 400,000 patients a year suffer from sudden cardiac death. Cardiac arrest is one of the leading causes of coma in the United States. Cardiac arrest results in significant decrease in blood flow to the brain. If the cardiac arrest is brief, the amount of brain damage may be limited. However, more prolonged episodes of decreased flow to the brain cause global and severe damage. Although the duration of time that results in brain damage is not well defined, significant damage can occur within minutes. In pathological studies there are different levels of damage seen, depending on the length of time of the cardiac arrest. With relatively brief periods the damage is restricted to the hippocampus, the memory center of the brain; with longer periods of time the cortex or gray matter is damaged, but the brainstem is preserved, which leads to a vegetative state. With longer periods of decreased blood flow, the brain is globally damaged and may lead to brain death. The brain is unlikely to tolerate lack of blood flow for more than 5 to 10 minutes.

92. How can you determine recovery of brain function after cardiac arrest?

The duration of brain ischemia is generally a good starting point to help predict outcome. However, it is often difficult to determine the exact time of cardiac arrest. Therefore the duration of the cardiac arrest needs to be taken in conjunction with a neurological examination and possibly other studies before a determination of function can be made. Several important elements on examination can help in determining the prognosis to include motor response, the reaction of the pupils, eye movements, and blood glucose level on admission. A determination of neurological outcome, however, should not be made until 3 days after the cardiac arrest. Studies have shown that 90% of patients who are destined to awaken do so in the first 3 days. Patients awakening after 4 days had persistent neurological deficits. Patients awakening after 14 days had severe neurological deficits. However, even patients who seem to wake up from coma early seem to have some cognitive deficits.

Lowering body temperature (hypothermia) a few degrees has been proposed as a technique to preserve brain function after cardiac arrest as well as large strokes and head trauma. The theory behind the potential benefit of hypothermia is that cooling of the body, and specifically brain tissue, can lead to reducing the metabolic rate of cells and consequently the generation of substances that may be harmful. Cooling techniques over the years have evolved, and our understanding of the risks and benefits of such intervention have matured. In the early stages of hypothermia the technique was crude, and therefore maintaining a certain body temperature was difficult. The complications noted with hypothermia, including infections, irregular heart rhythms, and clotting derangements, were in some cases fatal. Two large studies in 2002 shed light on the potential benefits in patients who had cardiac arrest due to ventricular fibrillation. The cooling was achieved by ice packs, cooling mattress, and cold air. Although these studies had some differences in the timing of cooling, both studies suggested a more favorable outcome in patients who were cooled. In one study, 49% to 55% of the cooled patients had favorable outcome, whereas 26% to 39% of patients who were not cooled had a favorable outcome. Overall, there were fewer deaths in the hypothermia group than in the normal temperature group. Although cooling of patients after cardiac arrest from ventricular fibrillation has been encouraged, most hospitals have not implemented such intervention. Furthermore, although other types of cardiac arrests may benefit from such an intervention, randomized clinical studies are not available at this time to help determine the efficacy and safety of such treatment. Other neurological conditions may also benefit from cooling, but again data are not available at this time for physicians to implement a new intervention.

The occurrence of cardiac arrest is often times unforeseen by family members, especially in younger individuals. The psychological impact of such an event is potentially the biggest contributor to indecision about the next step. The doctors often are hesitant to give the "bad news," and the family cannot accept the potential loss of a loved one. Decisions about care should be made in an environment that fosters an exchange of information between the family and the medical team and for the medical team to work on documenting the medical and neurological progress of the patient until more definitive decisions can be made. One of the major difficulties in understanding the neurological impact of cardiac arrest on the patient is that many patients have motor movements and eye movements that can be misinterpreted as purposeful, when in fact these movements are simple primitive reflexes. The quality of life is an important consideration in any decisions that are made regarding care.

At the time of my hemorrhagic stroke, I suffered cardiac arrest. Initially, it was thought that perhaps my heart failure was caused by my stroke. After several tests, it was determined that the cardiac arrest was actually due to my hemorrhage.

PART FOURTEEN

Risk Factors

What are the major risk factors for stroke?

Should patients with recent stroke also get evaluated for underlying asymptomatic coronary artery disease?

More . . .

93. What are the major risk factors for stroke?

The risks for stroke are similar to those of coronary artery disease and include hypertension, smoking, diabetes, elevated cholesterol, (especially low-density lipoprotein), sedentary lifestyle, poor diet, advancing age, and obesity.

The risks for strokes are similar to those of coronary artery disease and include hypertension, smoking, diabetes, elevated cholesterol (especially low-density lipoprotein), sedentary lifestyle, poor diet, advancing age, and obesity. We cannot discuss all these topics in detail, but it is important that the reader gets an understanding of the importance of controlling these risks and available treatments. Although elevated blood pressure is on its own a significant risk factor for vascular disease, untreated hypertension acts synergistically with other factors to increase the risk of vascular events. For example, elevated cholesterol in addition to elevated blood pressure increases the absolute risk of coronary heart disease by 10% above the risk seen with high blood pressure but without elevated cholesterol. There is another 10% absolute increase in the risk if smoking is added to hypertension and elevated cholesterol.

Elevated blood pressure: Elevated blood pressure is the number one cause of stroke, accounting for approximately 150,000 strokes per year. It is estimated that over 50 million Americans have hypertension. Although more patients are now receiving treatment for hypertension, approximately one third, most patients receiving antihypertensive treatment are not adequately controlled. Older patients have higher risk of having hypertension and lifetime risk of developing hypertension is 90%. It is clear from large population studies that hypertension contributes to an increase in death from heart disease and stroke. It is estimated that for every 20 mm Hg rise in the systolic (top number) blood pressure and for every 10 mm Hg rise in the diastolic (bottom number) blood pressure there is a doubling of mortality from cardiovascular and cerebrovascular disease.

Over the years our understanding of the contribution of elevated blood pressure to vascular disease has evolved and the values of safe blood pressure parameters have changed. New classifications for blood pressure lower the values of acceptable and safe blood pressure. Normal systolic blood pressure is considered less than 120 and diastolic less than 80. "Pre-hypertension" is defined as systolic blood pressure 120 to 139 and diastolic of 80 to 89, whereas hypertension is defined as systolic blood pressure of 140 to 159 or higher and diastolic of 90 to 99 or higher. If lifestyle changes do not improve the elevated blood pressure, the use of medications in those who are classified as hypertensive may become necessary. By adequately controlling the blood pressure, the risk of stroke maybe reduced by 35%.

In treating hypertension, it is best to have a multipronged approach, including weight loss, decreasing the intake of sodium (found in table salt), limited alcohol intake, and walking and/or exercise. Medications can be introduced if lifestyle modifications fail. Often, more than one drug is necessary. Many agents are available for blood pressure control, and it is best to discuss this issue with the primary care physician.

"Metabolic syndrome": This disorder was first described in 1988 by Reaven. It was noted that in some individuals, elevated lipids (cholesterol, triglycerides), high blood pressure, and elevated blood sugar often coexisted. This combination of risk factors contributes to an increase risk of developing vascular disease. The components of the metabolic syndrome include, in addition to the previously listed risks, obesity, a tendency to form clots, and increased level of inflammation. Inflammatory state as measured by C-reactive protein has been shown to be associated with elevated risk for vascular disease. The increased clotting tendency is in part related to increased levels of inflammatory proteins released by fatty tissue.

Elevated cholesterol: Cholesterol is an essential substance for proper integrity of cells in the body. Cholesterol can be divided into "good" cholesterol and "bad" cholesterol. High-density lipoprotein (HDL) is considered the good cholesterol and carries low-density lipoprotein (LDL), or bad cholesterol,

Risk Factors

away from the arteries. LDL forms the essential element of atherosclerosis. Atherosclerosis can be localized and forms into plaque. Atherosclerotic plaque is a complex of several different changes in the wall of the artery. The changes are initiated by penetration of the LDL cholesterol into the wall of the artery, which triggers macrophages (scavenger cell) and smooth muscle cells to begin to digest the LDL cholesterol. This initial step in engulfing the LDL cholesterol triggers chemical changes, which in turn attract more cells to react to the presence of LDL. Over time, this reaction results in disruption of the normal organization of the arterial wall, and slowly the plaque enlarges to narrow the artery. Narrowing of the artery disrupts the usually smooth blood flow, which may result in formation of clot. The narrowing may also simply reduce the blood flow, causing a stroke. However, although the enlarging plaque may be contained in the wall for a period of time, ultimately the plaque may rupture through the wall. This plaque rupture can cause an acute blockage of the artery and rapid clot formation, resulting in a stroke. This same process occurs in other arteries, including the arteries supplying the heart.

There have been many studies demonstrating the benefits of low LDL cholesterol in reducing the risk for all types of vascular events. Reducing the level of cholesterol could result in the prevention of 146,000 strokes per year. Initial studies looked primarily at the benefit of low LDL in the prevention of heart attacks. There was a clear relationship between the rates of heart attacks and the level of LDL cholesterol—the higher the LDL, the higher the risk of coronary heart disease. For example, an LDL level of 190 mg/dL increased the risk by almost fourfold compared with an LDL of 40 mg/dL. Another way to look at this is that every 30-mg/dL decrease in LDL resulted in a 30% change in the risk of coronary events. Although this is not direct evidence that similar reductions in LDL will help reduce the risk of stroke, the evidence was encouraging and suggested that perhaps similar benefits can be seen with stroke. Furthermore, because it is equally important to prevent heart attacks, which in turn can prevent stroke, the use of cholesterol-lowering drugs was hailed as an important advance in the treatment of vascular disease. Many people, however, were skeptical about the universal benefits of these drugs. In the past few years, data from clinical trials using different types of cholesterol-lowering drugs, known collectively as statins, have emerged to support the aggressive lowering of LDL cholesterol in all patients with recent vascular events or who are at high risk for vascular events. There have been more than 16 clinical studies that demonstrated the benefits of lowering LDL cholesterol. In 2004, the American Heart Association issued guidelines that recommended lowering the LDL in high-risk patients to below 100 mg/dL. But studies also demonstrated that lowering LDL below 70 mg/dL showed even more benefits and in some cases appeared to reduce progression of coronary as well as carotid atherosclerotic lesions. A more recent study, SPARCL, published in 2006 reaffirmed the benefits of lowering LDL with a cholesterol-lowering drug known as atorvastatin. In this study the risk reduction of stroke was significantly lower in the treatment group than in the placebo group. The benefit, however, was not immediate. There was also a suggestion from this study that taking atorvastatin had a beneficial effect in neurological outcome once the patient had a stroke. Although dietary changes may help lower cholesterol, many patients are not able to lower the LDL sufficiently or quickly enough to help prevent secondary events. At this time, the recommendations are for patients who are at high risk of vascular events to be treated with statins with a goal of lowering LDL below 100. There is also significant evidence to suggest that statins not only lower the LDL cholesterol but also have beneficial effects on the endothelium, the lining of the arteries. This benefit may be equally as important in the prevention of strokes and heart attacks. It is this benefit that has also sparked interest in studying statin therapy for other diseases, including vasospasms after subarachnoid hemorrhage, multiple sclerosis, and dementia.

Risk Factors

155

Statins have been reported to cause muscle damage, liver abnormalities, and muscle aches. Also, excessive lowering of cholesterol may cause intracerebral hemorrhages. The data on these potential complications suggest that for the most part these issues are somewhat exaggerated. In the most recent SPARCL trial, the number of patients who complained of muscle aches was similar in both groups, 5.5%. Muscle weakness was reported in 0.3% in both groups, and severe muscle damage known as rhabdomyolysis was reported in 0.1% in both groups. Elevation in liver function tests was higher in the group taking atorvastatin than placebo, 2.2% versus 0.5%. This elevation of liver function can be monitored by simple blood tests. As for the increased risk of intracerebral hemorrhage, this issue does not appear to be a prominent side effect of the treatment. From all the clinical trials that reported intracerebral hemorrhage with over 47,000 patients enrolled, a total of 160 intracerebral hemorrhages were reported in the statin groups versus 132 in the placebo group. In statistical terms these differences are not significant. However, even if the use of statins to lower cholesterol contributed to some of these bleeds, the benefits still outweigh the risks.

Smoking: Smoking is a major health care concern that clearly contributes to the development of vascular disease. Smoking cessation can lead to the prevention of 90,000 strokes per year. The effects of smoking on the arteries have been studied extensively, and it appears that smoking influences the elasticity of the vessel, damages the lining of the vessel (the endothelium), hinders natural repair mechanisms, increases the level of inflammation, and promotes clot formation. Smoking at any level seems to be a significant risk factor that when combined with other risk factors, such as diabetes and hypertension, can lead to a significant increase in the risk of vascular events.

Diabetes: Type II diabetes is clearly a major contributor to risk of vascular disease. Often this condition coexists with other conditions, such as obesity, hypertension, and elevated cholesterol. Elevated levels of blood sugar are often over-looked until patients present with symptoms or begin to have vascular problems. Hyperglycemia, elevated sugar, can promote vascular disease by augmenting the effects of elevated cholesterol on the lining of the vessels. Hyperglycemia also hinders the abilities of the body to repair damage in the arterial wall due to the lack of normal metabolic function. The diagnosis of diabetes may necessitate a special test known as "glucose tolerance test."

94. Should patients with recent stroke also get evaluated for underlying asymptomatic coronary artery disease?

It is clear that patients with strokes or carotid disease are at high risk of other vascular events such as heart attacks. Some studies have demonstrated that a significant number of patients with stroke have silent heart attacks and that approximately 16% to 37% of patients with carotid disease have at least one significantly diseased coronary artery.

Similarly, some patients who present for the first cardiac surgery can have coexisting asymptomatic carotid narrowing. In addition, patients with peripheral vascular disease (disease in the arteries supplying the legs) have been shown to have coexisting carotid and coronary artery disease. In a series of patients with peripheral vascular disease it was shown that narrowing of the arteries exceeding 50% was found in approximately 60% of patients. Significant asymptomatic coronary artery disease was found in approximately 25% of patients. Whether all patients with transient ischemic attacks or stroke need to be evaluated for underlying disease of the coronary arteries is not clear. However, primary care physicians can determine the risks of coronary artery disease in individual patients after a stroke and decide on the need for additional testing. Because stroke or transient ischemic attack is a marker of other vascular disease, an aggressive approach to treating all known risk factors should be undertaken in all patients.

PART FIFTEEN

Recovery and Rehabilitation

What is constraint-induced movement therapy?

Are there medications that can affect
recovery from a stroke?

What if normal swallowing does not return?

More . . .

A comprehensive rehabilitation program is the most important element in stroke recovery. However, rehabilitation is most effective when initiated as soon as possible after the stroke. Many patients achieve significant benefits in the first 3 months after the stroke. Although improvement may still occur after the initial 3 months, that improvement may be less impressive. Regression of recovery, however, is common as patients become "comfortable" with their deficits or when they are sent home after an aggressive rehabilitation program with no further outpatient rehabilitation. In the following months, many patients may begin to experience stiffness in the limb and pain that limits their ability to exercise. Side effects of medications may impact their ability to participate in exercises, and depression may influence the ability of the patient to engage in social activities.

Many studies have demonstrated that recovery occurs in a large part due to activation of several different parts of the brain, including the opposite side of the damaged brain in addition to areas of the brain that are usually not activated in a nondamaged brain. Some of this activation persists for many months, whereas in many patients a restricted area of persistent activation remains. It is still unclear how this activation contributes to potentially better or worse outcome in strokes. However, these studies clearly demonstrate the flexibility of the brain in response to injury with possible activation and inactivation of certain pathways to help unlock the ability of the brain to recover. Understanding these mechanisms may help us provide better treatments to improve the prospects of recovery.

Some rehabiltation hospitals have special programs geared toward younger patients, whereas other hospitals are interested in new rehabilitation techniques and research protocol.

Finding a rehabilitation hospital that fits the needs of the individual patient is very important. Some rehabilitation hospitals have special programs geared toward younger patients, whereas other hospitals are interested in new rehabilitation techniques and research protocols. Getting referrals from friends and family is a good way to start the search for a rehabilitation facility. Another way to learn about available rehabilitation hospitals in your area is to ask the doctors and nurses and case manager or social worker. Most importantly, and if possible, ask a friend or family member to visit the facility before the transfer. All rehabilitation hospitals have physiatrists and rehabilitation doctors, who will be involved in the care. Rehabilitation hospitals are also staffed by internal medicine physicians who can provide input regarding routine medical care. If a complicated neurological or medical problem arises during the rehabilitation, the facility can transfer you to an acute care hospital.

We were told to 'shop' for a rehabilitation hospital the same way we would approach buying a home. Once stabilized, I considered it essential to begin rehabilitating my body. I wanted nothing less than a full recovery; that was my goal. During my rehabilitation, I felt like I was having another stroke, and I was sent back to the acute care hospital for another five days of tests. When it was clear I was stabilized, I returned to rehab to continue the hard work. The therapies for stroke recovery are tedious and painful. Sometimes, it felt like the obstacles were insurmountable, but I persevered. Ten years post stroke, I continue to work to achieve wellness. I participate in clinical trials for stroke, I work with a personal trainer to keep strong, and most important, I keep a positive attitude, which is vital to sustain improvement. Stroke recovery proceeds at a snail's-- s-l-o-w --pace, but it is imperative to not give up.

95. What is constraint-induced movement therapy?

A few years ago reports emerged regarding a new treatment approach where part of the rehabilitation following a stroke included constraining the good limb for a few hours a day for 2 weeks. Small randomized trials have demonstrated conflicting results regarding the benefits of this intervention. The initial enthusiasm was probably premature as subsequent studies began to cast doubts on the initial observations. Therefore for now rehabilitation is best done in a center that is familiar with the latest approaches to treatment and staffed by dedicated individuals who can implement any rehabilitation protocols to improve the well-being of the patient.

96. Are there medications that can affect recovery from a stroke?

Human and animal studies have demonstrated that certain drugs can influence levels of neurotransmitters or chemical messengers in the brain. Drugs that have a negative influence on recovery and are commonly used in the treatment of patients after stroke include phenytoin and phenobarbital to treat seizures, benzodiazepines such as alprazolam to treat insomnia or anxiety, haloperidol used to treat behavioral disturbances and insomnia, and clonidine and prazosin used for treatment of blood pressure. Other drugs have been shown to have a positive influence on recovery, including methylphenidate and antidepressants such as paroxetine. These drugs with positive influence on recovery have been shown to augment the activation of the motor and sensory areas. The chemical effects of these drugs on neurotransmitters such as dopamine and serotonin may be important in activating residual or alternate pathways.

97. What if normal swallowing does not return?

Nutrition is extremely important to help the patient recover. Often, proper nutrition is hindered by the inability to swallow, drowsiness, behavioral issues, or recurring illnesses. Measuring certain nutritional parameters such as albumin and ferritin and following a patient's weight help to determine the nutritional status. Often, because of swallowing difficulties a modified diet is introduced, but if swallowing reflexes are impaired, other feeding methods need to be implemented. If swallowing reflexes do not improve in the initial few days after a stroke, then nutrition can be provided temporarily by nasogastric tube. If swallowing does not improve in the following 2 weeks, a gastric tube may need to be inserted. Although inserting a gastric tube is more invasive, requiring a minor operation, the procedure is safe. Ultimately, the gastric tube is safer, more comfortable, and more effective than a nasogastric tube. Unfortunately, approximately 75% of patients may continue to require feeding through the gastric tube due to lack of improvement in swallowing reflexes. The insertion of a gastric tube is sometimes considered by the patient and family as being an aggressive measure of maintaining nutrition in someone with severe disability. These issues are very complicated to address here. However, as is the case with complicated "life and death" decisions, it is important to consider the wishes of the patient first and then evaluate the medical information to decide on the appropriateness of any procedure that may prolong life at the expense of quality of life. In circumstances where the patient and family are unable to decide on the issue of gastric feeding, it is best to err on the side of feeding while awaiting recovery.

98. What is spasticity?

It is not unusual for patients who suffer from weakness as a result of stroke to develop spasticity on that side. Spasticity is the result of loss of the ability of the brain to maintain appropriate muscle tone. When the stroke destroys part of the motor circuit, the appropriate input and feedback mechanisms that provide just the right amount of tone are now malfunctioning in favor of increased tone. Some believe that this increased tone is a programmed survival mechanism that helps us to maintain our ability to stand and crudely grasp after suffering from a stroke. Unfortunately, this spasticity can stand in the way of recovery; it is painful and can cause severe joint problems. There are no easy cures for this problem. Muscle relaxant medications such as baclofen and Flexeril are used but are sedating. Some people use these muscle relaxants at night to help alleviate the discomfort. Botulinum toxin (Botox) has been injected in the affected muscles of a spastic limb, often with mixed results. Botox is most beneficial in

Recovery and Rehabilitation

patients who have spasticity caused by abnormal contraction of small muscles. For example, Botox may be useful in alleviating spasticity in the fingers but is less useful when used to alleviate spasticity in the whole limb. In the future it may become possible to insert probes in the brain that provide a small amount of electric current to allow us to change the balance back in favor of normal tone or more acceptable tone. Physical therapy and regular exercise on the affected limb are important to prevent some muscles from dominating the function of the limb and to help prevent joint and limb pain. A brace on the affected limb may also help prevent certain contractions.

Spasticity is a condition I have suffered since the onset of my stroke. It not only is painful, but quite annoying. Besides great discomfort, spasticity causes me to lose my balance and fall frequently. My left hand lacks small motor control, and my limbs on the left side are so tight with tone. It's like my left side is always in a state of tension, like tensing for a fight. My brain has lost the ability to let my left side relax. I do alternative therapies like acupuncture and deep tissue massage regularly to alleviate the pain and tension. These therapies provide relief, but it is usually temporary. I have done Botox in many areas—foot, leg, arm, shoulder—and it helped. Over the years, however, my body adjusted to the shots and they became less effective. Kinesio taping is a wonderful non-invasive relief that can be done by trained therapists. I also do serial casting on my leg and foot to stretch the tendons over a period of time.

99. Is irritability and depression common after stroke?

Stroke survivors go through an emotional roller coaster, including irritability, heightened level of anxiety, fear, and depression. Some people become obsessed with the possible risk of recurrence of another stroke to the point that they cannot function on a day-to-day basis. Worrying about recurrence of stroke is normal to some extent, but keeping this anxiety under control is important for recovery. In some patients it may become necessary to use treatments from meditation to medications. Talk about these concerns with friends and family, your physicians, or a stroke support group. Mood disorders are often seen in patients after a stroke. Many patients become depressed and anxious. They become withdrawn, less active, sleep is disrupted, they cannot focus or concentrate, and they are easily irritable. It has been shown that patients with right brain strokes are more likely to develop these problems, suggesting that this is the result of disruption of certain connections. Another explanation to these mood changes is that this is an expected reaction after such a loss of function. Many stroke survivors go through the five stages of grief: denial, anger, bargaining, depression, and acceptance. A patient needs to reach acceptance fast to help recovery. Depression may need to be treated with medications to improve recovery.

Depression is the most common psychiatric complication after stroke. The exact incidence is unknown, and the risk factors that lead to depression are not well defined. Risk factors that seem to be more common in those with stroke include the lack of a support system and living alone. Some studies have suggested that older patients were more likely to develop depression, but other studies demonstrated that younger patients are more likely to suffer from depression, especially in the early stage after a stroke. A comprehensive study using recognized depression scales was published in 2003. In that study, different degrees of depression were recognized nearly in 84% of patients. After the acute phase and during the follow-up phase, a year after the stroke 54% of men and 27% of women continued to have some degree of depression. The degree of functional impairment was associated with a higher risk for depression. This study also demonstrated that cognition of patients with stroke was affected by depression. The data suggest that depression is a frequent occurrence in patients after stroke. Early recognition of symptoms is an important element in any treatment of stroke. Controlling depression helps to improve the chances of recovery. The treatment of depression

Recovery and Rehabilitation

with antidepressants classified as selective serotonin reuptake inhibitors is important to initiate when deemed appropriate.

Stroke recovery is overwhelming. There are so many areas to reha-bilitate. I was always a very happy, good-natured person, but post stroke I had to start taking an antidepressant. My stroke caused severe motor control issues as well as some cognitive deficits. Prior to my stroke, I was a successful manager working in the software industry. I also cared for my three-year-old son. Stress was part of my life and I could handle it with ease, but after my stroke, stress would intensify all my impairments to the point where I have difficulty functioning. Post stroke, I couldn't take care of my own personal needs, let alone my child's needs. I lost all self-sufficiency and apparently went through an identity crisis. I could no longer work. My stroke robbed me of my computer abilities and my mul-titasking capacity— something I excelled at as a working mother. Now, I can only single task; I have difficulty focusing on more than one task at hand. I can no longer filter noise to focus on one sound. Initially this was so severe, that I could not have a radio or television on in the background if someone was talking to me. Naturally, the impairments of stroke would be cause enough for depression, but it was more than the ability to cope. The extensive brain damage altered the chemical balance in my brain. Clearly, I needed some synthetic help. As well, the tremendous frustration of lost independence exacerbates the level of irritability a stroke survivor experiences.

100. How are decisions regarding extent of care made?

Ethical issues regarding the care of patients with major medi-cal problems are to some extent expected. However, the most difficult problems that sometimes arise are conflicts among family members and conflicts with physicians. It is not un-usual to see different levels of expectation from different members of the family. It is also not unusual that different physicians may have differing expectations and sometimes differing opinions about the condition and treatment options available for a given patient. These issues create an environment for miscommunication, mistrust, and conflicts. This problem is especially prevalent in the first few hours or days after the occurrence of a devastating medical condition. The best approach for the family is to discuss the issues of care among themselves and to designate a spokesperson who can communicate with the medical team. This approach is likely to avoid some of the confusion that may arise from transmission of information through family and friends. Similarly, it is important for the physician to keep the family updated regarding occurrence of major medical problems, opinions of specialists, and progress. In making decisions regarding long-term care it is best for the family and the physicians to set aside personal preferences and biases and try to make the best decision based on the patient's wishes and reasonable predictions regarding the potential for recovery.

Recovery and Rehabilitation

Closing Remarks

I hope the information in this book has helped the reader acquire the basic knowledge necessary to promote understanding of the basics of stroke management. The book was written in the hope that patients and physicians can start communicating using common language. I also hope that the book shed some light on the complex nature of medicine. The great accomplishments in medicine fall short of a full cure for stroke, but the progress made in the past 15 years will certainly be surpassed by advances in the next 15 years. The great contributions made by medicine are only possible because of the willingness of patients to participate in clinical trials and to contribute not only their time but also their financial resources. Following is a list of resources that are available for stroke survivors. If you are so inclined, support groups for stroke survivors and their families can be found at many local hospitals.

Resources

American Stroke Association: 1-888-4-STROKE (1-888-478-7653). You will be able to obtain general information about stroke prevention and treatment.

National Institutes of Health: www.nih.gov. This website is full of up-to-date health information and lists of clinical trials and discussions of current research.

National Institute of Neurological Disorders and Stroke:

NINDS
Building 31, Room 8A-16
31 Center Drive, MSC 2540
Bethesda, MD 20892
301-496-5751
www.ninds.nih.gov

National Stroke Association:
9707 E. Easter Lane
Centennial, CO 80112
1-800-STROKES (1-800-787-6537)
www.stroke.org

Glossary

A

Aneurysm: outgrowth of an artery and rarely a vein, with a potentially weakened wall, that may bleed.

Arterial–venous malformation (AVM): abnormal collection of arteries and veins that can bleed.

B

Basilar artery: a major artery supplying the back of the brain formed by the merger of the two vertebral arteries.

C

Carotid arteries: two arteries in the front of the neck supplying most of the blood to the anterior part of the brain.

Cavernous angioma: vascular malformation that can bleed or cause transient ischemic attack-like symptoms.

Circle of Willis: connections of arteries inside the brain between arteries from the left and right as well as the anterior and posterior circulation. These connections help maintain flow in case one of the arteries is blocked.

Coiling: placement of metal coils in aneurysms to prevent the aneurysm from bleeding.

Computed tomography (CT): a fancy x-ray machine that takes pictures of the brain.

Computed tomography angiography (CTA): noninvasive test that uses a CT with intravenous injection of dye to visualize the arteries and veins in the body.

D

Dissection: separation of the layers of the arterial wall, causing narrowing and potentially resulting in stroke. This condition can occur spontaneously or with trauma.

E

Embolic stroke: This refers to stroke from blood clots or other debris that has traveled from another source before it finally gets lodged in an artery, causing stroke.

H

Hemorrhagic stroke: damage to the brain related to bleeding.

Hemorrhagic transformation: occurs when an ischemic stroke becomes hemorrhagic.

Heparin: blood-thinning medications that can be given intravenously or subcutaneously.

I

International normalization ratio (INR): blood test done to evaluate the effects of blood thinning of warfarin. The higher the INR, the "thinner" the blood. An INR of 1.0 is normal, meaning no effect of warfarin.

Ischemic stroke: damage to the brain related to obstruction of artery.

L

Lacunar stroke: stroke related to the small arteries in the deep parts of the brain.

M

Magnetic resonance angiography (MRA): uses MRI technology to look at arteries and veins.

Magnetic resonance imaging (MRI): uses a large magnet instead of an x-ray to see the inside of the body.

S

Spasms: constriction of the blood vessels, usually in reaction to inflammation or damage to the artery or chemical changes in the surrounding area, as may occur with subarachnoid hemorrhage.

Statins: class of cholesterol-lowering drugs.

Stent: tubular metallic mesh that is inserted inside of a narrowed artery af-ter the artery undergoes dilation with a balloon to maintain patency.

Stroke: any damage to the brain or spinal cord caused by obstruction or damage to artery or vein.

Subarachnoid hemorrhage: bleeding on the surface of the brain related to trauma or aneurysm.

T

Thrombotic: This refers to clotting of blood within arteries or veins.

Transcranial Doppler (TCD): an ultrasound used to evaluate flow inside the head.

Transient ischemic attack (TIA): transient neurological symptoms related to disruption of blood flow to certain parts of the brain.

V

Vertebral arteries: two arteries in the back of the neck that merge to form the basilar artery to supply the brainstem and the posterior part of the brain, including the occipital lobes and parts of the temporal lobes.

W

Warfarin: generic name for Coumadin, a blood-thinning medication that acts by inhibiting vitamin K and results in "thinning" the blood.

Index